CONSTRUCTING
RSI

DR YOLANDE LUCIRE works as a forensic psychiatrist in Sydney
and, occasionally, overseas. She has worked in prisons and in the
country and is Conjoint Senior Lecturer in the School of Rural
Health at the University of New South Wales.

CONSTRUCTING RSI

BELIEF AND DESIRE

Yolande Lucire

UNSW PRESS

A UNSW Press book

Published by
University of New South Wales Press Ltd
University of New South Wales
Sydney NSW 2052
AUSTRALIA
www.unswpress.com.au

National Library of Australia
Cataloguing-in-Publication entry:

Lucire, Yolande.
  Constructing RSI : belief and desire.

  Bibliography.
  Includes index.
  ISBN 0 86840 778 X.

  1. Writer's cramp - Social aspects - History.
  2. Somatoform disorders - Social aspects - History.
  3. Medicine, Industrial. 4. Medical anthropology. 5. Social epistemology. 6. Medical care - Evaluation. I. Title.

  363.1109

Printer BPA
Cover image Dana Lundmark

CONTENTS

FOREWORD

Pain, distress and impaired function are common symptoms which bring men, women and children of all ages, shapes, sizes and creeds seeking at least alleviation, if not a diagnosis or explanation for what ails them. For some, the diagnostic answer is immediately evident and the diagnosed condition is amenable to a proven therapy or, perhaps, a medication, a course of physical or occupational therapy, a surgical procedure, avoidance of an offending precipitator or another change in a specific behaviour. The efficacy of a particular therapy has usually been derived by application of the scientific method.

In many instances, however, the cause will not be evident, and this negates any chance of designing of a suitable therapy. When it is not possible to unequivocally link a specific cause with an explanation, symptomatic treatments are often applied. The impact of this medical activity extends far beyond individuals and their immediate families both in well-understood conditions and in those in which ignorance still reigns.

Repetitive strain injury (RSI) is a not uncommon diagnosis that falls into the category of being an ill-understood condition with impacts and ramifications far afield.

In this book, Yolande Lucire tackles RSI from many interesting perspectives. As a psychiatrist, she has used her extensive study of an afflicted patient population diagnosed with 'RSI' in Australia to take the reader on a journey that begins by laying a broad and general background of important concepts.

These early chapters provide the reader with necessary scaffolding of background from which Dr Lucire then brings into sharper and more detailed focus her analyses of RSI from several perspectives. The book concludes with case examples, which add to the texture and richness of the work.

The author's thesis is that RSI cannot be explained from a patho-physiological or biomedical perspective. Rather, she uses a vantage point of one seeking to understand how exploration of a condition such as RSI can clarify some of the paradoxes in behaviour of doctors and society.

An analysis of the RSI pandemic is at the core of this work and in the detailed chapters Dr Lucire examines the historical perspective as well as industrial and professional considerations.

This is a scholarly piece, one that has multiple dimensions.

I commend this work not only to those interested in RSI as a per-plexing phenomenon but also to those who wish to allow their mind to explore territories that one might not ordinarily expect to emanate from studies of RSI, a condition which remains a conundrum to many a patient, employer and doctor alike.

S. Bruce Dowton
Dean, Faculty of Medicine
UNSW

PREFACE

On 8 April 2002, President Bush set out his Ergonomics Plan, launching an initiative to protect workers from job-related repetitive-stress injuries. He wanted to see the development of voluntary industry-safety guidelines and to monitor how companies adopted them. Administration officials unveiled a four-point plan to help industries with high rates of muscular–skeletal injuries to begin developing guidelines during the next six months to prevent neck strain, carpal tunnel syndrome and other ailments caused by repetitive tasks. Officials of the Occupational Safety and Health Administration said that they would bring enforcement actions against industries that had high injury rates and took few actions to reduce them.

On 9 December 1996, a federal jury awarded more than US$5 million to one plaintiff for repetitive stress injuries (RSI), also known as carpal tunnel syndrome. The case centred on the claim that Digital Equipment Corporation, the manufacturer of the keyboards, was aware of the risks of using their product and failed to provide proper warnings. This case, tried before Judge Jack Weinstein in the U.S. District Court in Brooklyn, awarded $5.3 million to one plaintiff and about $700 000 total to two more plaintiffs. This is believed to be the largest RSI award and the first major victory in keyboard litigation in the United States.

In the United Kingdom, 28 February 2002 was declared to be International RSI Awareness Day. The Trade Union Council's figures showed that one in every 50 workers was suffering from the symptoms of RSI. It claimed that, in 2001, 5.4 million days were lost in sick leave due to RSI and, every day, six workers left their jobs forever because of RSI.

On 23–24 February 2002, the *Weekend Australian* displayed a photograph of a young nail technician, Ms Downey, with her six-month-old baby. The New South Wales State government had successfully prosecuted her employer, a beauty parlour owner, in the NSW Chief Industrial Magistrate's Court for $37 754.37. NSW WorkCover had sought fines and legal costs over repetitive strain injuries suffered by a hair stylist and two nail technicians. The workers had complained about their conditions and had claimed that they did repetitive work for 12-hour days without a break.

A spokesman for WorkCover said that, although the injuries occurred in 1998 and 1999, the issue of repetitive strain injury had been brought to the salon's attention in 1996.

Well before all that, in 1986, the Australian disorder, RSI, was identified as yet another episode of epidemic occupational cramp, craft palsy, a disorder classified in the *International Classification of Diseases* of the World Health Organization within the Mental and Behavioural Disorders section. RSI is mass psychogenic illness, masquerading under a myriad of diagnostic attributions, several of which are applied to each case. Physical entities do not affect the mind: only frightening beliefs about them do. Occupational tasks, keyboards, posture, overwork and overuse do not cause RSI. Rapid movements, repetitive work, static strain, discomfort, ergonomics do not cause it, nor does any physical element to which it is attributed. Epidemic RSI is caused by the belief that all or some of these have the capacity to harm the body.

This information was brought to the attention of the readers of the *Medical Journal of Australia*, to WorkSafe Australia, to WorkCover, and to the courts. The journal failed to retract seminal papers that had introduced RSI. Prominent in their citation base were publications endorsed by Australia's peak medical advisory body, the National Health and Medical Research Council (NHMRC) and the National Occupational Health and Safety Commission, WorkSafe Australia.

Two kinds of knowledge were operating: that created over long periods by scientifically minded researchers, and that held up by the power of institutions, experts and judicial decisions.

I wanted to draw attention to the medical opinions and legal actions that created RSI, in order to answer my critics who suggested that I was saying, 'It's all in your mind, dear.' I was forever trying to explain that these are painful illnesses but their symptoms are not traumatic in origin, nor are they injuries in any known sense of that word.

Judges who see causation as a matter of common sense use their power to apply an attribution. Causes do not just come before — they bring about effects. Causes are identified by using the science of epidemiology and are subjected to testing by scientific method. Junk science thrives in Australian courts and those who write about its absence have not made inquiries from experts.

Doctors transmit beliefs, but cannot make people give them up. Belief is governed by desire.

Trade unions wanted to protect workers' interests but, instead of offering immediate help to their members to deal with their workplace problems, they told members who called for help to go to the doctor. The trade unions failed to recognise that they were handing over their traditional responsibilities to the medico-industrial complex. By doing so, they almost made themselves redundant.

A search of World Law discloses a further 225 papers advising of legislation, all of which has been promulgated on the assumption that RSI has physical causes and is preventable by physical means. These regulations promote the unvalidated beliefs that cause the symptoms of the epidemic, functional disorder. The terms 'RSI, injury' throw up more than 22 000 Internet web sites devoted to the prevention, identification and treatment of this condition, which is assumed to be a traumatic injury.

Twenty years on, epidemics of RSI continue to follow prevention campaigns.

This book started as a PhD thesis, *Ideology and Aetiology: RSI, an Epidemic of Craft Palsy*. I want to thank my supervisor and intellectual guide, Professor Randall Albury, at the School of Science and Technology Studies at the University of New South Wales, the Wellcome Trust for the History of Medicine in London, the late Roy Porter and Bill Bynum, who read early drafts, and my examiners, Edward Shorter, Arthur Kleinman and Stephanie Short, who legitimated my position. I am grateful to John Rowe, who insisted it should be published, UNSW Press for being so persuaded and my editor, Carl Harrison Ford, for making it comprehensible. I am grateful to my extended family, to my friends and colleagues who encouraged me.

I particularly want to thank the scoffers as they forced me to reproduce all these orthodox, unoriginal, well-established, conventional ideas in an environment where the whole world seemed to be out of step with them. I also apologise those who recognise their words and ideas represented here, as many references that were cited in the thesis had to be left out of this book.

The author can be reached at lucire@ozemail.com.au.

ABBREVIATIONS

ACOA	Administrative and Clerical Officers' Association
ACTU	Australian Council of Trade Unions
AMWSU	Amalgamated Metal Workers' and Shipwright's Union
APSA	Australian Public Service Association
ATO	Australian Taxation Office
CTD	Cumulative trauma disorder
CTR	Carpal tunnel release
CTS	Carpal tunnel syndrome
DPO	Data processing officer
DSM	Diagnostic and Statistical Manual of Mental Disorders
EC	European Community
EMG	Electromyography
FCU	Federated Clerks' Union
GP	General practitioner
ICD	International Statistical Classification of Diseases and Related Health Disorders
NHMRC	National Health and Medical Research Council
NIOSH	National Institute of Occupational Safety and Health
NOHSC	National Occupational Health and Safety Commission, also called WorkSafe Australia.
OCBD	Occupational cervico-brachial disorder
OHSU	Occupational Health and Safety Unit
OOS	Occupational overuse syndrome
PSB	Public Service Board
RCT	Rational choice theory
RSI	Repetitive strain injury
TUC	Trades Union Congress
VDU	Visual display unit
VTHC	Victorian Trades Hall Council

INTRODUCTION

LOCATING RSI IN THE MEDICAL LITERATURE AND DIAGNOSTIC SYSTEMS

Mean motives will probably be ascribed to me,
for I am presenting the history of a scandal.

David Joravsky, *The Lysenko Affair*

The 'new' industrial epidemic disorder of symptoms in the arms that was known in Australia as 'repetitive strain injury', 'RSI', 'occupational overuse syndrome' or 'OOS' and 'teno' has previously been reported in the medical and other literatures in both sporadic and epidemic forms as 'writers' cramp', 'occupation neurosis' and 'craft palsy'.

Occupational cramp is classified as a 'mental and behavioural disorder' in the section on somatoform disorders at F48.8 in the *International Classification of Diseases* of the World Health Organization. Cramp involves disturbances in both function and sensation and it has long been recognised as signalling conflict about work.

The expressions 'cramp' and 'craft palsy' are commonly used to refer to the problem and they seem to be the briefest, least pre-emptive and least value-loaded terms available. They have been used interchangeably throughout this book to describe the affliction. Not entirely comprehensive descriptions, they have the advantage of being more succinct than 'functionally impaired manual occupational capability'.

Transient cramp, discomfort and local fatigue are universal phenomena experienced by all of us. The similar symptoms that are the subject of this book persist well beyond the time tiredness and injuries take to recover, for months or years. The functional disorder causes work disability on a massive scale.

Since it was first recognised, the syndrome has been classed as a 'functional' disorder in neurological, psychiatric and occupational health textbooks. The term 'functional' implies the absence of an organic disease base and this suggests psychogenesis, which is causation by ideas and emotions and having its origin in the mind. In both physiology and sociology, 'functional' refers to a process driven by its consequences and it implies lack of disadvantage. The afflicted in this epidemic were having, sociologically speaking, 'functional', that is culturally approved reactions. They were able to get on with their lives with financial support that would otherwise not have been available to them.

The epidemiology of RSI suggests that, in the absence of a set of legitimating beliefs, those afflicted in this epidemic would not have suffered pain. They might have made their decisions about whether or not to go on working using pragmatic considerations. The opportunity to claim and to suffer was the consequence of a political definition of illness that was not in accordance with rationalist or medical science.

The injury theory of RSI was an example of Lysenkoism, a truth sustained by officialdom, supported by powerful institutions yet, at the same time, the discourse was not meeting any of the criteria for science.

Thomas Kuhn, in his seminal text, *The Structure of Scientific Revolutions*, introduced the concept of the paradigm, an organising principle that can govern perception itself. The book itself started a revolution in the evaluation of competing theories in the physical sciences. Among other things, Kuhn told us that a paradigm was a pre-scientific set of ideas that comprised the beliefs of a given society and passed for 'common knowledge'. Paradigms are frequently ideological in content.

A paradigm is the knowledge that members of a scientific community share and, conversely, a scientific community consists of those people who share a paradigm. A prevailing paradigm will determine the direction of research.

What Kuhn called 'normal science' proceeds through a process of paradigm shifts because, as knowledge grows through scientific endeavours, information that does not fit the existing paradigm becomes available, and the paradigm becomes, as it were, wobbly at the edges. A new paradigm, a new theoretical framework, is introduced to accommodate inconsistencies.

Scientific methodology is based on generating hypotheses and testing them to see if they can be falsified; indeed, this methodology is what distinguishes science from other fields of human inquiry. The statements constituting a scientific explanation must be capable of empirical test, as the criterion of the scientific status of a theory is its falsifiability, or refutability, or testability (Popper 1963).

Two incommensurable paradigms of explanation guided diagnosis and management of the Australian epidemic of arm symptoms. These were the injury paradigm and the somatization paradigm.

In the injury paradigm, symptoms were seen as evidence of a musculotendinous injury caused by a preceding task or by various characteristics of the workplace. A person was seen as a physical body, of brain, tissue and muscle, damaged by trauma inherent in manual tasks and workplace conditions. The epidemic was to be managed by control of traumatising agents and the subject, usually female, was not to be held responsible either for her condition or for her recovery. This paradigm was focused on the body of the subject and its interaction with the physical environment (Mathews & Calabrese 1982).

The injury paradigm, described in detail in this book, claimed the dominant position on the moral high ground.

The notion of RSI, or overuse, interested unions and industrial activists who sought to control output and protect jobs threatened by word processors which, as steel nibs and typewriters had done, seemed to threaten job security. The unions wanted to have medical justification for so doing. The high moral standing of the physicians who became involved in providing this justification was borne out by their zeal and high-minded contribution to a campaign of preventive medicine and workplace improvement. RSI was promoted by unions and accepted by government because, being ideologically based, it served social functions which were considered legitimate at the time.

The epidemic of RSI is better explained as somatization than as injury. The somatization paradigm interpreted undiagnosable symptoms as functional disorder or, if a pathological entity was known to have preceded their onset, as functional overlay.

However, to say that a claimant was somatizing, or suffering from a somatoform disorder, one would have to disregard the social implications of the patient having been given a diagnosis of RSI. To say that a cramp subject was somatizing did not accommodate her rational or even irrational desires.

The diagnosis effectively ruled out any investigation of the ethical position of the somatizing subject as, for the duration of the incapacity, the physician assumed responsibility for the patient's illness behaviour and for the granting and taking of indulgences and exemptions.

Somatization theory focused on the vulnerable affected subject. It failed to accommodate the role of the physician in guiding the emergence and the succession of symptoms. It did not accommodate the societal and cultural factors that made somatizing an acceptable, even desirable, way of being in the world. While blaming the workplace, through diagnosing injury or medicalising the patient by diagnosing somatization, both formulations served the interests of the medical profession.

Defining somatization as a medical issue embodied the assumption that the patient was sick in some way that was accessible to medical intervention. However, it provided no remedies for the afflicted, nor did it articulate a means of avoiding such epidemics in future.

The epidemic highlighted the extent to which medical practitioners, all over the world, do not differentiate scientific knowledge from their personal beliefs. Doctors have little comprehension of why science might matter to them in their day-to-day healing activities and craft practices.

Baroness Wootton suggested that a distinction be made between 'what is treatable by medical means' and 'what doctors treat', that is, between what doctors do when they are behaving in the special fashion peculiar to their profession and what they do when they drop the Aesculapian mantle and behave as ordinary men and women. This distinction is extremely blurred, as every intervention is code-named 'treatment' and the activities of the medical profession are subject to confidentiality and mystification.

A history of how and why the epidemic arose has the greatest explanatory power and is much more informative than medical models of explanation. The identification of the medical and social causes of epidemic illness has been the enterprise of Ivan Illich (1974, 1975) and the Marxist sociologist Vincente Navarro (1976).

Those who wish to know more about details of case studies or methodology are referred to my thesis *Ideology and Aetiology: RSI, an Epidemic of Craft Palsy* (Lucire 1996), which is available in the library of the University of New South Wales.

1

SOME SOCIOLOGICAL AND PHILOSOPHICAL PRELIMINARIES

For each illness that doctors cure with medicine, they
provoke ten in healthy people by inoculating them with the
virus that is a thousand times more powerful than any
microbe: the idea that one is ill.

Marcel Proust (1871–1922)

It is axiomatic that medical activity has the goal of keeping a population healthy and preventing unnecessary ill health and disability. It is
precisely this axiomatic view that is to be examined in this book. The
RSI epidemic was, apparently, an exception to this rule. Harming
rather than healing as a result of medical intervention is a recognised
problem. The frequency with which this happens is a matter of concern to primary care physicians. In a monograph, *To Harm or to Heal*
(1981), the Royal College of General Practitioners warned that the
doctor could influence somatic fixation in a positive or negative way.
His treatment influenced how the patient would deal with his own
complaint.

Some studies have predicted the pitfalls of medical practice.
Australian medicine fell into these traps when doctors tried to
respond to the challenge of epidemic arm symptoms.

In 1951, Talcott Parsons wrote about the sick role and the complementary role of the physician. Freidson published on *The
Profession of Medicine*, his 1970 study of 'the clinical mentality'. In
1975, Ivan Illich developed a theory of iatrogenesis, causation of epidemics of illness by doctors, cultures and societies, all of which anticipated Scheff's 1978 analysis. Scheff revealed that it was

unacceptable for a physician to miss an existing condition but more acceptable to follow the 'better safe than sorry' rule and incorrectly diagnose a condition which did not exist. Vincente Navarro saw the development of the medico-industrial complex as serving the power structures in a capitalist society.

Patients, physicians, institutions and government all contributed to the epidemic of RSI by their diagnosis and management of this disorder.

THE PARSONIAN IDEAL

In 1951 Talcott Parsons conducted a case study of the practice of medicine in the Boston area, but he was unable to complete it. He described an ideal: how both physicians and patients were thought to act in the United States in the middle of the twentieth century. Parsons described four aspects of the sick role: first, patients were not to be held responsible for their condition; second, they could not be expected to get well by an act of will, as they could not help it; third, the sick patient was entitled to exemptions, such as staying home from work; and fourth, the patient was obliged to seek technically competent help and to co-operate with the physician in the process of trying to get well, as it was the sick person's condition, not his attitude, that needed to be changed.

Parsons saw that the sick role was a product of motivated action. He saw illness as a possible response to social pressures, a way of evading responsibilities. He recognised that the privileges and exemptions of the sick role were often desirable objects towards which the patient was positively motivated, by his account, 'usually unconsciously'. The institutions in society were thought to control motivation to recover (Wolinsky 1980).

Because they identify illness and supervise those defined as sick, doctors are expected to embody society's dominant values. The moral position of the sick person is not a consideration for a physician, nor is the moral position of a physician a concern for a patient. Refusal to define a person as sick under certain circumstances leaves that person open to social judgments such as being 'lazy, criminal or irresponsible' (Illsley 1980). The sick role is attractive, yet yielding to temptation is not considered blameworthy.

The profession placed great emphasis on its obligation to put the welfare of the patient above personal interests. Physicians were expected to be steeped in altruism as the medical world intended to

exclude both commercialism and the profit motive. While helpless-
ness, lack of technical competence and high levels of anxiety make
patients vulnerable, exploitation of the sick is in the realm of the
unthinkable.

The physician was expected to treat illness as an applied scientist
and in scientifically justifiable terms, just as today's physician is
expected to practise evidence-based medicine, dispensing those
remedies that have been demonstrated to be effective and refraining
from administering useless ones.

Parsons was aware that both patients and physicians deviated
from their idealised roles and he gave the matter consideration.
Perhaps like any social scientist whose research depended on the continuing goodwill of the researched group, Parsons did not suggest
any but the most vague reasons for such aberrations. A sociologist
could take the potential for exploitation for granted.

Neither of Parsons' idealised roles was evident in the RSI epidemic. There was no biological component to be changed: the
claimants' beliefs and attitudes were the problem. Those claiming to
be afflicted sought exemption from their normal responsibilities
largely because they were being made to feel entitled to do so.
Physician and patient had complementary roles, with the physician
providing technically competent help to a patient whose problem is
assumed to be accessible to medical intervention. The evidence in the
RSI epidemic was that a physician was selected, often after a search,
because he or she took a view of the symptoms consistent with that
of the patient and trade union. He was selected because he was recommended as someone who knew what to do, which was to remove
the worker from harm and provide a certificate for compensation. He
was not chosen because he promised to provide a cure. The physician
placed a patient in a sick role and relieved her of responsibility, as she
was henceforth only following orders. The worker was defined as
injured and, as such, was not responsible for what happened next.
The physician was unable to help yet was willing to indulge in a pas
de deux of doctoring activities, given and received. The patient
appeared to comply with the physician's instructions, while at the
same time she was both aware and not aware of their futility, knowing and not knowing at the same time.

According to the Ehrenreichs (1978), certain features of the
social construction of sickness were set up to discourage people from
using sickness as a way of dropping out. These barriers were lowered

in the RSI epidemic and a situation was engineered where becoming ill could provide a downright advantage.

FREIDSON

Eliot Freidson, a sociologist, stressed that he had no wish to deprecate the grandeur of medical discoveries: his analysis concerned the physician working in the community in the United States in 1970. Whereas Parsons had specified expectations, Freidson looked at physicians' performances and at the responsibility they had for illness, against the backdrop of illness as a social construction and defined, sociologically, as deviance.

Unlike Parsons, Freidson did not see the physician to be the legitimator of illness. Rather, he argued that medicine was engaged in the creation of illness as a social state. By virtue of being the authority on what illness 'really' was, the physician created the social possibilities for acting sick. He had the right to decide who was ill just as the priest established what was holy or profane and the judge adjudicated who was innocent or guilty.

By not holding the patient responsible, the physician provided a model for how others were to respond to a sick person. Patients were not encouraged to take responsibility for their illnesses, which had to be controlled and managed. Granting of the status of being ill, together with its attendant exemptions, could be made conditional on the patient's acceptance of treatment. The profession was then able to extract a toll in the form of unquestioned submission to the remedies that medicine had to provide. Patients knew they were expected to comply with treatment, if only to demonstrate that they were co-operating in their own recovery. The legal system demanded this proof and this trade in indulgences was widely exploited in the RSI epidemic.

Exemption from responsibility for working was assumed to be a consequence of the seriousness of the illness. The patient had no control over going to work, as the doctor made this decision for her. Granting exemptions involved a certain amount of circular reasoning, especially in those cases where the sick role was sought in the absence of physical evidence of a disease. Claimants cited the advice of their doctors to explain their absence from work and avoided revealing that they had selected doctors who, they had been reliably informed, would provide such certificates if they made certain complaints.

According to Freidson, Parsons' formulation did not take into account the fact that what patients did stemmed from what they understood to be the situation. So patients who genuinely believed themselves to be ill behaved as if they were ill, much the same as patients with biological derangements.

The genuineness of this belief was rarely at issue, only its scientific status and origins.

In Freidson's view, degradation ceremonies, submitting to examinations and the like, formally created secondary deviation (see also Garfinkel 1956). Reid, Ewan and Lowy (1991) described the reaction of women to getting a diagnosis of RSI and the examinations through which they had to pass with sceptical physicians. Although the afflicted women got the diagnosis they wanted and had their symptoms legitimated, their 'pilgrimage of pain' and their feelings about such procedures made a moving tale. Union activists sought to eliminate these difficulties and were successful in identifying and recommending physicians to whom complaining workers might go.

Where Parsons had ignored what people understood from their experiences with physicians, Freidson addressed what it meant to be ill. He was not concerned with what had caused the patient to be sick. He identified what he called 'secondary deviance', which involved the problems caused by a diagnosis and by being labelled sick.

Why people defined themselves as sick and why and where they decided to seek health care has been extensively researched before. In brief, the sick role becomes attractive to people who are anxious. It can resolve a conflict between attending to personal needs and obligations and going to work and earning an income.

THE CLINICAL MENTALITY

Freidson studied doctors as well as the patients and identified what he called the 'clinical mentality'. He found North American physicians to be crude pragmatists, not scientists. They looked at the world in clinical terms and their aim was not knowledge but action. Unsuccessful action and action for its own sake were both preferred over no action at all, on the assumption that doing something was better than doing nothing.

Medical practitioners were more likely to believe in the value of their actions than to manifest a sceptical detachment. They were more likely to believe in what they were doing in order to practise, to believe that they did good rather than harm and to believe that what they did made the difference between success and failure. They were prone to rely on what they believed to be results and to value their clinical knowledge and gut response above abstract principles and book knowledge. They were likely to tinker if they were not getting results by conventional means.

The physician would argue that he could not suspend action in an emergency simply because he was uncertain. He could invoke uncertainty, as it provided him with a psychological ground from which to justify his pragmatism. He could then extend action to less urgent situations. The physician could not afford to be sceptical of himself, of his experience, of his work or of its fruit. He relied on what he took to be probabilities and on his own senses. Unable to see what other physicians did, he was likely to overestimate his virtues and to consider himself as an expert in all human problems. Freidson quoted a sardonic comment: 'Clinical experience is frequently personal mythology based on one or two incidents, or on stories by colleagues'.

According to Freidson, the clinical construction of illness was influenced by the needs of the physician to believe in what he was doing, as he knew that if he believed that the patient would recover, this influenced the patient to respond favourably.

During the RSI epidemic, the opposite effect emerged: physicians were advised that the condition was resistant to treatment. They were swayed by popular opinion that the task was the cause. They removed patients from the assumed cause and influenced them to remain in the sick role for long periods.

Freidson adverted to the problems caused by bias. Their own patient populations lead physicians to assume that other populations are similar to those with which they have experience. Individualist in his orientation, each physician assumes personal responsibility for the way in which he manages his cases. He does so in a world prone to be self-validating and self-confirming. The roles of scientific knowledge and the opinions of others are minimised, as they bring their own practices into question. A physician reporting on his own poor clinical results legitimates an expectation of failure and this can lead other clinicians to expect the same. This can lower professional standards. Expectations, good and bad, can have a predictable effect on the health of patient populations.

In common with Thomas Szasz and Ivan Illich, Freidson decried the encroachments of medicalisation, pointing out that what have been called crime, degeneracy, lunacy, sin and even poverty are all being called illness. The medical profession established jurisdiction over illness and over anything to which that label might become attached. As a consequence, the established responsibilities of medicine extend far more widely than its demonstrated capacity to cure. The profession has been successful in putting the label 'illness' on many disapproved types of behaviour. In turn, the label carries with it the implication that the behaviours are properly, or even successfully, managed by physicians, as physicians show themselves willing to manage or deal with such problematic issues. The jurisdiction of medicine is elevated to legitimate the claim that the proper management of many forms of deviance is treatment in the hands of a skilled and responsible profession.

In a circular fashion, this leads to the illogical conclusion that the behaviour that physicians seek to manage must be an illness. This circularity has to be examined further.

THE PHYSICIAN AS A MORAL ENTREPRENEUR

In Freidson's analysis, the physician could also operate as a moral entrepreneur, an essential figure in the creation of those group events now known as moral panics. Becker (1963) described one type of moral entrepreneur, the 'rule creator', who is interested in changing rules because some evil profoundly disturbed him to such an extent that any means is justifiable to do away with it. He seeks to punish the evildoer.

In Freidson's account, moral entrepreneurs in medicine are commonly part-time practitioners who crusade in health matters. The thrust of their activity is towards political power as they seek to implement measures designed to improve what they see as public health. They give press interviews and testimony in court. They are often responsible for legislation. They want to place jurisdiction for their concerns in the hands of health professionals rather than leave them with society. Freidson identified lay interest groups sometimes led by, and always including, prominent physicians whom he described as '... the most flamboyant moral entrepreneurs of health, untrammelled by professional dignity, crusading against the menace of a specially chosen disease, impairment or disease-producing agent'.

Such moral entrepreneurs are essential players in any moral panic. As this book goes to press, some medical moral entrepreneurs are creating panics about the prevalence of depression, the disabling effects of anxiety and the consequences of child sexual abuse. Others seek to have professionals attend on people who have been exposed to both real and hypothetically traumatic events. Moral entrepreneurs invite attention to their proposed remedies, which, they claim, would surely cure. They see traumatogens, mental and physical, as being at the base of epidemic ailments, mental and physical. The currently dominant paradigm assumes that many of life's problems are caused by trauma. Farrell (1998) treats both posttraumatic stress disorder and the public's panic over child sexual abuse as cultural tropes, and explores the ideological interests that they serve.

Physician entrepreneurs are more likely to see the environment as more dangerous to health than does the layman and are more likely to emphasise the seriousness of the health problem preoccupying them by estimating the number of cases that have not yet been undiagnosed and therefore remain untreated. They are disposed to see mental illness where the layman sees nervousness, to see illness where the layman sees variations within the broad range of normality, to see a serious problem where the layman sees a minor one. They are biased towards the creation of sick roles; hence they produce an increase in the number of diagnosed cases of whatever it is that bothers them. They move the goalposts on levels at which blood pressure is to be considered treatable and the sugar level at which diabetes is to be diagnosed. They press their licence as physicians to manage the newly defined sick within their relevant specialty frameworks.

In brief, the medical profession is more prone to see illness and the need for treatment than it is to see health and normality. This selective perception is both self-confirming and self-sustaining.

Freidson cites Szasz (1961) and his effort to dissect the character of the newly emergent problem of the relationship of institutionalised expertise to the individual's right of to self-determination. He also anticipates Scheff (1978), who describes how the application of the 'better safe than sorry' medical decision rule promotes the multiplication of a possible mistake, the type II error.

A type I error is a false negative, a situation where a doctor fails to diagnose a disease. A type II error is a false positive, where a doctor diagnoses a disease or a condition that the patient does not have.

In Scheff's view, one of the norms of medical practice is how frequently a type II error is allowed to occur in medical procedures. Pressure not to miss a treatable condition results in investigations being ordered with increasing frequency and this in turn leads to escalation of health care costs. He argues that, when they occur too frequently, type II errors have more significant social and economic consequence, especially when they develop into a collectively noxious practice.

SCHEFF, DIAGNOSIS AND ERRORS

Thomas Scheff reported on the medical literature concerning iatrogenic, physician-induced disease and identified the process by which the physician unnecessarily caused the patient to enter the sick role. He recognised the tendency of medicine to dismiss iatrogenesis as 'due to quirks of particular patients', for example, as the consequence of patients' malingering, hypochondriasis or of exhibiting merely functional illness, in the sense of 'functional' for the patient. Scheff rejects this notion, which blames patients for their behaviour and takes the position that the cause of functional disease lies in the medical procedures themselves. He believes that most people obligingly come up with appropriate symptoms if the physician tells them that they are ill.

Scheff believed that most physicians learn early in their training that, like many important cultural norms, it goes without saying that it is more important to avoid judging a sick person as well than to judge a well person to be sick. Commonsense might suggest that it is not only culpable to dismiss a sick patient but also a bad economic decision. A sick person who has been misdiagnosed will not only seek treatment elsewhere but is likely to report his or her experience in the community.

This caveat is endorsed in both the current diagnostic schedules, the *International Classification of Diseases* (ICD-10) published by the World Health Organization in Geneva and the *Diagnostic and Statistical Manual* (DSM-IV) published by the American Psychiatric Association. These works caution against the diagnosis of hysteria or somatization for fear of missing a disease. That is, physicians who wish to make a diagnosis of functional disorder find little encouragement from the medical establishment to do so.

Scheff questioned the assumption that type II errors were relatively harmless. The logic of the 'better safe than sorry' rule rested on two assumptions: first, that an undetected and untreated disease would grow to a point where it 'endangered the life or limb [sic] of the individual' and, second, that medical (mis)diagnosis of illness was without consequences. He suggested that physicians guided by this medical decision rule place some patients in the sick role when they could have continued with work and their normal pursuits.

Lamenting the lack of empirical data for the prevalence and effects of type II errors, Scheff had to go back many years to cite Bakwin's 1945 study of physicians' judgments regarding the advisability of tonsillectomy for 1000 schoolchildren at a time when tonsillectomy was a fashionable operation. Of these 1000 children, 611 had already had their tonsils removed. Other physicians then examined the remaining 389 and 174 were selected for tonsillectomy. A third group of doctors was put to work examining the remaining 215 children and 99 of them were adjudged in need of tonsillectomy. Still another group of doctors examined the remaining children and nearly half were recommended for the operation. Almost half of each group of children was adjudged to be in need of the operation. Even assuming that a small proportion of children needing tonsillectomy were missed in each examination (a type I error), the number of type II errors in this study far exceeded the number of type I errors.

Scheff and Freidson shared some concerns about the bias of the profession towards the medicalisation of social problems. Scheff accepted the capacity of type II errors to harm where a diagnosis was erroneously made of a stigmatising psychiatric condition. That is, Scheff was more concerned that patients should not be labelled as having a psychiatric disorder when they did not have one, than if they were diagnosed incorrectly as having a physical disorder. This reluctance on the part of the medical profession to diagnose a mental disorder remains a problem. This, in turn, results from a lack of understanding of the concept of psychogenic, which refers to causation by ideas and emotions. In common language, psychogenic illnesses are called stress-related and in that formulation the population readily accepts them. When physicians fail to understand the concept and believe that such a diagnosis implies it is imaginary or in some other way non-genuine or associate it with mental illness, they feel constrained against making such a diagnosis. This reluctance to even consider emotional causes seems to be very strong and remains the reason for the profession's wholesale failure to diagnose conversion symptoms correctly.

The physician, reluctant to indulge in masterly inactivity, wants to do something, so he invokes pragmatism, saying that he has to start treatment in order not to waste time. However, there is little that presents as a symptom in the arms that is life threatening, so one might reassure the patient that it is possibly cramp before making a pronouncement on a physical diagnosis. The only life-threatening disease that presents in the arm is angina, the pain associated with heart disease. But the dominant ideology so powerfully governed medical perception in this moral panic that I have seen two patients in whom arm pain that turned out to be angina had been misdiagnosed, perhaps on certificates, as RSI.

Scheff argued that type II errors involved the danger of having a person enter the Parsonian sick role in cases where the illness could have been left unattended without incurring any serious consequences. The patient's attitude to his illness is usually considerably changed by the series of medical procedures. The seriousness with which a doctor views the patient's symptoms profoundly influences the course of a chronic illness. Scheff also believes that the medical profession does not take the consequences of inappropriate interventions seriously. Though occasionally mentioned in the literature, such adverse consequences to the patient's health have never been the subjects of a proper scientific investigation (see Balint 1957; Illich 1975). If this is the case, then this study of an accidental and natural experiment is indeed a rarity.

In 1979 Sissela Bok, an ethicist, criticised the use of placebos on ethical grounds, arguing that their prescription to unwitting patients illustrates two miscalculations: prescribers ignore possible harm and they fail to see how trivial gestures build up into collectively undesirable practices. She argued that resort to placebos may actually prevent the treatment of an underlying, undiagnosed problem. At the same time, the use of placebos results in immense costs building up for treatments whose benefits are transitory at best and ultimately wasteful of the trust a patient places in a physician. The placebo, then, is a resort of the poor diagnostician, of one who cannot grasp the concept that social stresses can make people sick in a very non-specific way.

Scheff's position is that physicians and the public all typically overvalue treatment in the face of uncertainty. He points to studies which show that people who go to the doctor are under considerable strain and tension and that they are extremely suggestible. Scheff recognised the difficulties associated with the research he saw as necessary, work which would include experimental studies into the extent to which misdiagnosis by physicians might determine the risks of unnecessary entry into the sick role.

The RSI epidemic was precisely such a situation. Had it been set up as an experiment and subjected to prospective scientific research it might have yielded a great deal more information than my surveys conducted through the perceptions of afflicted subjects and the records I created.

An application to perform such an experiment would not pass an ethics committee. For example, one might want to study the long-term effects on a population of getting a scare as a result of misinformation. One might want to raise a false alarm by telling the occupants of a building that its lift wells disgorged toxic fumes that caused harm. This experiment could not be done, as an ethics committee would not permit it. For good reasons, research cannot be conducted on people who are not aware that they are the subjects of an experiment. The idea that they may have been poisoned would cause the building's occupants to become anxious, to panic and to feel that they had the symptoms of having been exposed to toxic fumes. They would go to various doctors, some of whom who would confirm that they had been affected. This possibility exposes the risk that some cases of doctor-legitimated illness would occur in vulnerable people. Without doubt, these illnesses would have been psychogenic in that they would have been triggered by the misinformation contained in the false alarm. Some experimental subjects and their doctors would latch onto such an explanation for whatever symptoms they were experiencing at the time and they would continue to believe in false causes and to suffer beyond the time frame of the experiment. They might prove to be extremely difficult to cure, especially if a potential for legal action entered their agenda.

Lashford v Plessey was a significant NSW Supreme Court decision (1982) in an early RSI case. The judge decided that the employers had negligently failed to warn of the dangers of a harmless occupational task. The real danger lay in giving the warnings, which contained and transmitted the false beliefs that caused the psychogenic symptoms. A court insisted that employers act in a way that was known, by some, to be both harmful and unethical. Similar warnings to workers are still demanded by the Trades Union Congress in the United Kingdom and by the European Community in Brussels.

It is indeed a curiosity that a study researching the effects of making such warnings would fail to be granted funding on ethical grounds if it were presented to the National Health and Medical Research Council (NHMRC), as that institution played a significant part in the genesis of the RSI epidemic by promoting the false beliefs that caused it.

RATIONAL DIAGNOSIS AND TREATMENT

Karl Popper suggests that we need social theory to be able to predict the unintended consequences of our actions.

In 1982 Culver and Gert adapted rational choice theory and applied it to the practice of medicine. Rational practice in medicine was bound to be dictated by the beliefs, reasons, motives and desires of physicians and patients.

The notion of rationality has permeated philosophy from its inception. In its broadest interpretation, rational choice theory invites us to understand individual actors (which in specified circumstances may be collectives of one sort or another) as acting, or more likely interacting, in a manner such that they can be deemed to be doing the best they can for themselves, given their resources and circumstances as they see them. This template explains what people do (actions) to get what they want (desires), in terms of what they believe to be the case (beliefs). It examines how they explain why they did whatever they have done (reasons and conscious motives) and how they hide from themselves and others the fact that what they want is not acceptable and cannot be openly acknowledged (unconscious motivation). Rational choice theory takes into account how people prioritise all that they want (ranking of desires into a hierarchy). This all takes place in a situation where some behaviours are permissible and some are not (social norms) and people know what is considered good and what they can get away with (social values). Rational diagnosis is to be as free as possible from error. Rational treatment has the capability of eliminating or minimising the effects of a disease. It is also rational to expect that patients value health over illness, that iatrogenic harm is to be avoided and that pain, disability and work incapacity are undesirable and, in the terms of this theory, evils.

The activities of both physicians and patients, their beliefs and the reasons they offer for them and the conflicted or even perverse desires which they could not acknowledge have all been examined.

According to Elster (1994), in a rational world, actors (or in this case study, doctors and patients) would be expected to collect and consider all the relevant evidence for a course of action. In practice, the evidence a physician collects is determined by how much he really wants to know. If a doctor knows more, he might have to embark on a course of action that is to not to his or her advantage. Specifically in the RSI epidemic, if treating doctors had wanted to recognise the functional disorder, they could not have continued to do what they did to patients, collectively, to generate millions of dollars worth of medical costs in pursuit of treatment-resistant complaints.

Reasons are always conscious and occasionally glib, and always based in events in the past. A reason, for example, is how a person felt when he or she went to the doctor. This does not explain his or her motivation, which might have been to seek a cure or might have been to obtain a work disability certificate. When reasons are unconvincing and self-serving they are called rationalisations. Motives, expectations about the future, are more likely to both explain and cause actions than are reasons. A motive to punish an employer might be seen as altruistic in the hands of an activist, but the doctor cannot be permitted to involve himself in the battles of others, in a war that is, unfortunately, claiming victims. According to the *Oxford English Dictionary* definition, a victim is a person destroyed or injured that an object may be gained or a passion gratified. The use of the word 'victim' should alert a social scientist.

An irrational belief is one that is held by a person with sufficient knowledge and intelligence to know that it is false, is logically or empirically incompatible with a number of beliefs that the person knows to be true, and whose incompatibility is apparent to almost everyone with similar knowledge and intelligence (Gert & Clouser 1986). In Elster's view, one reason for holding irrational beliefs is failure to collect or acknowledge available evidence. Actors have many reasons for failing to inform themselves.

The responsibility that doctors have to hold rational beliefs is an ethical problem rather than a legal one. The ethical issue for a medical practitioner would be to decide how much he or she wanted to take into account before dealing professionally with a patient.

RATIONAL TREATMENT PLANNING

A rational treatment plan is one that deals with the scientific data as well as with what is 'for the good of the patient' (Wulff 1976). Sometimes the doctor is asked for a medical certificate at a time when the patient's predicament motivates her to need time off. At the same time, the certificate sacrifices her reputation for good health. This can place the doctor in a conflict, one that is resolved if the doctor knows to consider the health of the patient to be his priority, over and above her predicament or need for time off or money. In brief, a medical certificate should be a truthful account of the patient's illness and, in the case of compensation, its causes.

Rational action involves three optimising operations: finding the best thing to do, which depends on what we believe, on what we want to do and what is expected of us; examining the evidence; and collecting the right amount of evidence to justify both what we believe and what we want to do. The beliefs we settle on are determined by what we desire. Or as the philosopher David Hume suggested: 'Reason is and ought to be the slave of the passions'.

Elster's analysis of how and why rationality does not always prevail could provide a template for the history of events in the RSI epidemic. Much can be gained from an examination of reasons and motives as well as beliefs and conflicted desires of everyone involved.

CONTAGION OF BELIEF AND BEHAVIOUR

The most parsimonious view of epidemic hysteria is that there are only two essential elements: the availability of a belief and the understanding that certain behaviours have certain consequences (Kerckhoff & Back 1968). When an epidemic of hysteria involves the body, the soma, it is called an epidemic of somatization.

This view of hysteria, as behaviour based on beliefs and opportunities, raises the question as to whether somatization should automatically or even legitimately be seen as a medical condition. Hysteria, at least in its epidemic form, is generally considered to be functional rather than dysfunctional for many of those affected.

Western medicine places somatization within the jurisdiction of the medical establishment. If somatization is indeed the product of beliefs and opportunities, then one might examine what should or, more notably, should not be done about it.

Somatizing patients are constantly in peril of misdiagnosis, hence mistreatment. Care needs to be taken with somatizing patients, as they are not immune to disease. They are far more likely than the rest of the population to have health impairments that cause stress. Poor health, in turn, manifests as a general state of weakness ready to be moulded in accordance with the expectations of doctors and patients. Their disease might merit attention for itself or for the anxiety it is causing.

In *Theory of Collective Behaviour*, Smelser (1962) defined collective behaviour as mobilisation on the basis of new belief, one that redefined social action. The simplest form of hysterical belief was defined as 'one empowering an ambiguous element in the environment with a generalised power to threaten or destroy'. Hysterical beliefs are unverified rather than untrue. Flight and panic are expected behaviours as people try to escape from the threatening elements. If, however, a positive element is introduced, alleged to have power to reverse the negative outcome, then the belief in it becomes a wish fulfilment belief. Smelser called such a positive element a 'gimmick'.

As people make an effort to acquire this means of salvation, the behaviour associated with avoiding the threat becomes a craze or fad rather than a panic. Smelser believed that the adoption of hysterical beliefs involved short-circuiting, in that the explanation for the stressful situation was sought not through a logical process of considering alternative explanations, but by jumping immediately to a high level of generality involving preconceptions of causality and seizing upon some explanation at this level to make sense of the felt strain. He pointed out that, while such explanations might be accurate, they were unlikely to be.

In the case of RSI, the newly defined hysterical belief was that occupational tasks had the capacity to cause injuries. By offering relief from the hazard in the form of a compensated sick role, doctors could offer their patients safety from the newly defined hazards. The physician, by adopting the belief, was able to provide the wish-fulfilling belief. In this way, doctors promoted the gimmick, the positive element with the power to reverse the negative outcome. They became the vectors of the epidemic.

In 1968 Kerckhoff and Back studied an epidemic of hysterical contagion based on a belief that an insect, dubbed the 'June Bug', had been imported in cargoes of fabric and that its bite caused certain discomforts. Participation in this outbreak was seen as functional for many of the women involved, particularly those who were unable to face or even admit to the existence of other stress in their life. They did not document the stress affecting the women in their case studies.

Adopting the belief that the June Bug was the cause of their symptoms provided some objective explanation for the women's amorphous sense of discomfort. Although noting that the belief had a functional (in the sense now of positive) aspect to it, Kerckhoff and Back also stressed its negative impact, namely that a fear of a toxic bug represented the addition of a new source of strain to the environment. Their explanation did not cast negative aspersions on the individuals involved.

Kerckhoff and Back saw contagion of beliefs as a rapid dissemination, a less rational process than diffusion. They pointed out that the actor must already know the consequences of the available action and it must be attractive but previously discouraged by some kind of constraint. As the belief spreads, people report their symptoms at an earlier stage and others become sensitised to notice such symptoms and their increasing prevalence and legitimacy. Kerckhoff and Back recognised that the unconscious played a role, but only in so far as the motive to adopt the sick role was not acknowledged. Symptoms were automatic and authentic physiological responses to increased levels of strain. There was a widely accepted cause, so resistance to adopting illness behaviour was lowered.

Kerckhoff and Back traced information about the June Bug through friendship networks. Modern hysterias are transmitted through the media and affect susceptible people who have never met and who usually cannot identify where they first came across the beliefs that governed their behaviour and experience. Social norms changed for the period of the RSI epidemic. Social pressure brought about conformity with a new norm, one that deemed a new form of behaviour, escape from hazard, to be appropriate in just such an ambiguous situation. Workers entered the sick role and the compensation system on behalf of symptoms that they would not have attended to before. Participants in social interaction apparently understand many things, even though such matters are not mentioned explicitly (Cicourel 1973). New norms and behavioural contagion altered the judgment of the gatekeepers who regulated entry into the compensable sick role, as well as that of doctors and tribunals. This change in norms had massive consequences on absenteeism and on the costs of workers' compensation.

MEDICINE AS A MORAL ENTERPRISE: KENNEDY

Ian Kennedy, a lawyer, questioned how medicine was thought and practised (Kennedy 1981, 1988). He examined what he called 'the real face of medicine' and concluded that medicine was a moral enterprise. In his view, doctors used power to determine what was and what was not legitimate illness and they did so with varying degrees of consent from patients. He also argued that doctors interfered in matters that they could not affect.

Kennedy reasoned that unquestioned jurisdiction over the determination of what was and was not an illness and who should and should not occupy the sick role gave doctors unlimited power in this domain. It turned medicine into a political enterprise favouring certain interests. The social institution of medicine was there to persuade us that our preoccupations had to be related to medical matters and to doctors who, alone, had the competence to define them in medical terms. Interplay between illness and morality followed, played out on a political and social plane. The sick role, being ill, became a status, not a state, granted or withheld by those who had the power to do so.

Kennedy reminded us that before the advent of modern medicine some of the conditions now regarded as illnesses were attributable to possession by evil spirits. He pointed out that the notion of possession has not fallen before the onslaught of scientific medicine but has been retained, in that the body of an ill person is now suspected of being possessed by disease, even where the only evidence for physical disease is a complaint of ill health. He pointed out that, while using the rhetoric of medicine, doctors made decisions based on no more than their personal values. Kennedy asked the questions: What is a medical decision? What decisions are within a specific competence of a doctor to make? What is it appropriate for a doctor to decide? Are there decisions which should not be made by doctors alone?

Kennedy saw that the doctor encouraged the process whereby he was seen as the purveyor of panaceas. Even though doctors would be the first to deny having any, it was gratifying to their perception of themselves as helpers, as it guaranteed they would never cease to be wanted. Quite simply, it gave doctors power.

Kennedy reported that he was constantly confronted by doctors complaining, often quite rightly, that they had to make too many difficult decisions it was not their job to make, that they were expected to do society's dirty work and that they needed guidance. The moment Kennedy tried to offer guidance or suggest what should be done, however, he was immediately met by a chorus of cries, all variations on the theme that these were medical matters after all and that he should not trespass on matters of professional competence and judgment.

Although Kennedy did not endorse the conclusion of Ivan Illich, he echoed Illich's opinion that medicine was a moral enterprise in that it defined what was normal and proper in behaviour. Medicine had acquired the authority to label one person's complaint a legitimate illness, to declare another person sick though he did not complain, and to refuse such recognition to a third.

Kennedy suggested that we were forced to the conclusion that a doctor's unique competence extended from management of a broken leg to the management of our comfort and happiness and our social wellbeing. He pointed out that the moment this debate was opened, so too were the floodgates of vitriol. He maintained that he was not trying to criticise doctors, but 'I am trying to analyse what I think is a reality and what produces that reality'. He thought it unfair that responsibility in many areas of human concern has been improperly shifted onto doctors by the rest of us, simply because doctors seemed prepared to take it on and because others were happy to have them bear this responsibility.

The RSI epidemic was an illustration of the position taken by Illich, namely that the medical establishment has become a danger to health. Professional mystique hid the fact that doctors were partly responsible for a large amount of the ill health they claimed to cure. Illich popularised a technical term, iatrogenesis, for the new epidemic of doctor-made disease. It is composed of the Greek words for physician or healer (*iatros*) and for origins (*genesis*). The conflict between the medical health care system and patients appears as iatrogenesis and it manifests itself in three forms.

It is clinical iatrogenesis when pain, sickness and death result from medical care. Clinical iatrogenesis comprises conditions for which remedies, physicians or hospitals are the pathogens or sickening agents. It includes damages inflicted with the intent of curing or exploiting a patient, as well as actions pre-emptively taken by the doctor to cover him against a potential malpractice suit for failing to cover every eventuality.

It is social iatrogenesis when health policies reinforce dependency and ill health. This refers to the medical reinforcement of a morbid society, one which exponentially bred demand for the patient role. It is structural iatrogenesis when medically sponsored behaviour and delusions restrict the autonomy of people by undermining their confidence in growing up, caring for each other and aging.

Cultural iatrogenesis is the deeper, structurally health-denying effect of the profession in so far as it destroys the potential of people to deal with their weaknesses in an autonomous way.

Illich recognised the doctor as a pathogen alongside resistant strains of bacteria, hospital corridors, poisonous pesticides and badly engineered cars. He claimed that the proliferation of medical institutions, no matter how safe and well engineered, unleashed a social pathogenic process. Over-medicalisation changed adaptive ability into passive medical consumer discipline.

The prophesies of Illich were writ large in the RSI epidemic, in the first years of institution-building and the early years of the medicalisation of occupational health.

Illich's view was that iatrogenic disease comprised only that illness 'which would not have come about unless sound and professionally recommended treatment had been applied'. That is to say, iatrogenic illness was a consequence of what apparently passed for sound and professionally recommended treatment. Within this definition, patients could sue their therapist (or employer) if he or she had not applied a recommended treatment and which in itself carried a risk of making them sick. Illich (1975) continued:

> Most malpractice does not fall within the categories of having acted against the medical code, incompetent performance or dereliction out of greed or laziness, but most damage occurs in the ordinary practice of well trained men and women who have learnt to bow to prevailing professional judgment and procedure, even though they know (or could or should know) what damage they do.

Illich further warned: 'The damage done by medicine to the health of individuals and populations is very significant. These facts are obvious, well documented and well repressed.'

In his critique of Illich, Vincente Navarro (1976), an American Marxist thinker, saw iatrogenesis as a symptom or byproduct of the struggle between the powerful classes and the less powerful workers. In his explanation, responsibility for iatrogenesis did not lie with the medical profession at all, but with the powerful corporate classes that had a dominant influence in health care delivery institutions, in governments and in insurance agencies. By judicious use of incentives, this class ultimately controlled the parameters within which doctors did their daily work.

Navarro (1976) argued that the prime roles of the medical profession involved keeping the workforce healthy so that greater profits might be generated for employers, and also mystifying people as to the real causes of illness in the world, creating, in Marxist terms, a false consciousness. Navarro's somewhat unpopular views of medical practice have been amply demonstrated in the history of the RSI pandemic.

2

DISEASE, ILLNESS AND SOMATIZATION

'Illness' [stands] for what the patient feels when he goes to the doctor and 'disease' for what he has on the way home from the doctor's office. Disease is something an organ has; illness is something a man has.

Edward J Huth (1976)

THE DEVELOPMENT OF THE CONCEPT OF SOMATIZATION

The concept of somatization plays an important role in contemporary clinical theory and practice. It is a name given to a process usually referred to by the layman as 'emotional' (Lucire 1990). Somatic symptoms without apparent cause have been categorised in many different ways: neurosis, hysteria, functional overlay, illness behaviour, abnormal illness behaviour, ideogenic illness, psychogenic illness, functional disorder, stress induced disorder, nothing at all wrong and hypochondriasis. Some of these terms are antipathetic, some hostile, others empathic or, at best, ambivalent and, like much psychiatric terminology, value-laden and judgmental.

The term somatization came out of psychoanalytic theory (Stekel 1943) and it does not carry the same pejorative connotation as the others. It can be used in the transitive tense. 'What is it that you could be somatizing?' This can be taken to mean: 'What is making you sick? Is your body trying to tell you that you are worried about what to do and you have to make a hard decision?'

Somatization is a major concern in Western medical practice, as somatizing patients are often hospitalised and they attract invasive diagnostic and surgical procedures as well as arduous medical treatments which are costly, fruitless and sometimes lead to serious iatrogenic disease (Kirmayer et al. 1991).

According to Fabrega (1990), the concept of somatization does not extend to other societies. However, emotional causes for illness are recognised everywhere. The patient would often agree to understand that the symptoms are, in common parlance, 'stress-related'. Cures are underpinned by the notion that an authority, such as a physician or other healer, is then able to change the somatizing patient's understanding of his or her body, which is what healers of psychogenic illness do. They ameliorate the illness experience and provide reassurance about expectations where possible. Many societies would not encourage physicians to become involved beyond diagnosis and evaluation of somatizing patients.

Patients who have to pay their doctors do not so readily indulge in treatments they know to be useless. The term rich hypochondriac belongs to a period when it cost a lot of money to be sick. Where a third party pays, treatment-seeking behaviour becomes more affordable and more common. Where medical resources are in short supply, doctors prioritise treatable conditions. Where medical personnel and resources are in surplus, physicians expand their domains.

In standard Western medical theory, the body is understood in anatomical, physiological and biochemical terms. Untoward changes (including those caused by trauma) are termed disease and are identified through their clinical manifestations; these, in turn, are supported by physiological, biochemical and radiological deviations from roughly agreed upon norms (Canguilhem 1947). Diseases have symptoms and signs, do not change much between subjects and cultures and can be recognised from textbook descriptions. The extent to which a person is upset when sick is also expected to conform to culturally agreed-upon norms for the disease in question.

Somatoform symptoms, those without justifying disease, can sometimes be diagnosed from their own characteristics. For example, angina is usually felt in the central chest, whereas da Costa's syndrome, the emotionally caused mimic, the cardiac neurosis, generally presents with left-sided chest pain, in accordance with the known position of the heart. In today's language, it is a stress-related symptom. The sufferer is relieved to know he is not having a heart attack and he welcomes the diagnosis. Somatoform symptoms do not follow established patterns but are consistent with what the patient believes about the state of his body (Engel 1970). They may involve motor and sensory modalities at the same time. Such a combination is seen only rarely in clinical medicine, occasionally in multiple sclerosis and sometimes in peripheral neuropathy. A patient with those disorders may be very sick indeed and clinical signs are much in evidence.

Ill health, illness experience and illness behaviour become standardised in a culture. When a patient's response to a disease differs from a prevailing norm, the contemporary physician may invoke the concept of somatization. The patient might be in too much distress, might be in distress for too long, might be presenting symptoms that cannot be accounted for in terms of that disease or might not be responding to treatment. The physician may address the social, psychological and cultural factors that have influenced the patient's illness experience and behaviour. To do so, he completes his examination, dons his metaphorical white coat of authority and says to the patient words to this effect: 'I cannot find any physical causes for your symptoms. Is there something the matter?'

Individuals whose illness behaviour does not conform to majority norms might be said to somatize. Minority social or ethnic groups have different norms of illness expression that often do not conform to those of the dominant group. The concept is accordingly evaluative, culturally and socially laden and extremely vulnerable to changes in both physicians' and patients' norms and expectations. Somatization incorporates a value judgment, but remains a discernible phenomenon.

There are physicians who decline to follow these well-established principles. They invent novel diseases or follow those who have done so. They mount campaigns for their acceptance. As the lay community is not educated in the scientific basis for the corpus of medicine, followers of fringe ideologies are seen as leaders in their field and attract a following. They do so by creating an impression that their explanations are at the forefront of medical research, that they are just about to find a cure and that their knowledge is superior to that in textbooks: in brief, that they know what they are talking about. The personal characteristics of charismatic doctors are not well recognised. Their days would be numbered if they were to be asked to quantify their successes, to practise evidence-based medicine or to oblige courts with the scientific basis for their beliefs.

THE CONCEPTS OF DISEASE AND ILLNESS

Philosophers have developed an extensive literature on the key concepts of illness and disease and the subsidiary notions of sickness, impairment, handicap and disability (King 1975; Kräupl-Taylor 1976, 1980; Margolis 1976).

The rest of the medical profession is confused. In 1986 Merskey, a psychiatrist, suggested 'that what doctors treat can be accepted as disease provided that we recognise that the significance of disease must vary with circumstances'. His view informs the debate. The definition fails and must fail because it is entirely circular, yet it cannot be ignored as it is precisely this view of illness and disease that passes for common knowledge and forms the rationale for the interventions of doctors into all spheres of life. Kendell (1975) warns that any definition of disease that boils down to 'what patients complain of' is worse than no definition at all, as disease is free to expand and contract with changes in social attitudes and therapeutic optimism and is at the mercy of idiosyncratic decisions by doctors and patients. Moreover, equating illness with complaint allows the individual to be the sole arbiter of whether he is ill.

Kräupl-Taylor, a psychiatrist, attempted to measure illness by quantifying morbidity, physician–patient contacts, costs and incapacity. His medicocentric position is that disease is 'what medical personnel are willing to treat'. This definition confers power onto the physician and is dependent on subjective feelings and judgments.

A clinician, Jeremiah Barondess, cut across the philosophical problem with a linguistic solution: he suggested that the terms disease and illness should refer, respectively, to the biological component and the state or status of the sufferer (Barondess 1979).

Disease consists of untoward changes in the body, identified at macroscopic, microscopic and molecular levels and is characterised by changes, by disruptions in the structure or function of a system. It may be due to a variety of causes, may persist, advance or regress and may or may not be clinically apparent.

Illness, on the other hand, is a human event, an array of discomforts and dislocations resulting from interactions of a person with his body and with his environment. The stress may be a disease, a stressful series of life events or a perceived threat that is symbolic.

Barondess points out that in 50 per cent of clinical contacts, illness lacks a definable biological basis.

> Disease and illness are not congruent and each exists in the absence of the other. The capacity of physicians to interfere in any fundamental way with the natural history of diseases is relatively new, so their efforts have traditionally been directed towards the amelioration of the discomforts, fears and concerns of their patients, that is, to the illness experience.

Illness, so defined, is congruent with somatization, symptoms whose form is determined by beliefs and cultural expectations. Somatization accounts for symptoms that are superfluous to the diagnosis of the specific disease, or symptoms unsupported by the specific clinical signs that would permit diagnosis of a disease. Somatization can be a response to a disease or to the belief that one has a disease, in so far as it represents a threat to security. In simple terms, symptoms of illness can be caused by the very fear of having a disease.

A disease, the belief that one has a disease and the experience of having a disease are all translated into an idea, one that has implications. A person then feels and behaves in accordance with what he or she would do if afflicted with the condition that has been diagnosed. To demonstrate: if your father dies and you do not know about it, you will not grieve. If you are informed that your father has died (and he has not), you will grieve, even though he is still alive. It is not the fact of your father's death but the belief that it has occurred that causes the mental state of grief. Similarly, if a person has been told, albeit mistakenly, by an authority, the doctor, that he or she has a disease, he or she will worry, will feel unwell, and will do what the doctor says, just like the person who actually has that disease. The authority to diagnose disease confers great responsibility onto doctors.

THE BACKGROUND TO THE CONCEPT OF SOMATIZATION

William Cullen was generally credited with coining the term 'neurosis' in the eighteenth century, when it signified a disturbance of the nervous system, affecting sensation or motion. The neuroses, which were described at the back of textbooks of neurology, comprised clinical states whose manifestations could not be attributed to identifiable neurological lesions, together with those for which no pathophysiological basis could be found. Hysteria was the prototype.

In 1837 Benjamin Collins Brodie, a surgeon with an extensive practice concerned with bone and joint disease, wrote of hysteria: 'It is not the muscles which refuse to obey the will, but the will itself which has ceased to work'. He held the opinion that 'at least four fifths of the females who are commonly supposed to labour under diseases of the joints, labour under hysteria'. Brodie's remarks were consistent with contemporary notions of conflicts of will and desire, which underpin the diagnosis.

In England, Robert Brudenell Carter's *On the Pathology and Treatment of Hysteria* (1853) informed the concept of hysteria. He argued against the biological model, urging that hysteria's real aetiology was to be found in the patient's inability to deal with emotions. Anticipating Freud by 30 years, Carter dramatically changed the understanding of hysteria. He identified three causal factors: the temperament of the individual, the event or situation that triggered the attack, and the degree to which the subject was 'compelled to repress the exciting causes'. In Carter's view, these included sexual passions, hatred and envy. According to Carter, complicated hysteria generally involved moral and intellectual as well as physical derangement. Carter also believed that emotion could produce serious disorders by acting on muscular, vascular and secreting organs. He wrote that the influence of emotion was greatly increased by local and general debilitating agents and by circumstances that made an individual body part the subject of attention. Because these derangements were much more common in the female than the male, Carter believed that the woman was not only more prone to emotions but also 'more frequently laboured under the necessity of trying to conceal them'. Carter lamented that: 'If the laity could be made to understand the essentially simulative character of complicated hysteria and the amount of moral delinquency involved in it, they would accede readily to all demands for full control over unhappy victims'.

Influenced by Carter, Sir John Russell Reynolds wrote in 1869 that some conditions of paralysis as well as disorders of function and sensation depended upon a morbid condition of emotion, of an idea combined with an emotion, or by an idea alone. These conditions could last a long time, could simulate complex neurological (or any other) disease and could disappear entirely on removal of the erroneous idea. He separated these conditions from insanity, hysteria, hypochondriasis and malingering, and he published separately, again, on writers' cramp (1878).

In 1873 John Paget elucidated the volitional aspects of hysterical paralyses, also noting that the conflict of desires led to palsied inaction: 'They say, "I can not". It looks like "I will not" but it is "I cannot will".'

By the time Dr William Gowers published his two-volume *Manual of Diseases of the Nervous System* in 1888, most neurological entities were classified as they are today. As pathological detail has become available at various levels of complexity, a mere handful of diseases and lesions have been winnowed out from the syndromes caught in the early twentieth century concept of 'neurosis'.

During the reign of Jean Martin Charcot at the Salpêtrière, a hospital in Paris, the predominant and most dramatic form of the neuroses was *la grande hystérie*. Charcot's well-tended specimen patients were able to reproduce its manifestations, contortions and fits, at will and for monetary gain, many years later. Charcot's reaffirmation of a neurological theory was said to be part of an attempt to gain greater professional recognition for neurology, which at that time incorporated psychiatry. His official explanation was that hysteria involved a brain disease with functional peripheral manifestations (Briquet 1859). In private, Charcot insisted that the origins of the phenomenon were sexual (Gay 1988).

Pièrre Janet also reported on the moral aspects of hysteria, but he saw their relationship to medical concerns quite differently from Carter. He expressed concern about the admonitions of moralistic physicians (Janet 1925).

Janet proposed a more parsimonious explanation than that of Charcot, with the notion of the *idée fixe* at the basis of each patient's disorder giving rise to symptoms in each case (Janet 1901). Sexuality was implicated in only four instances in Janet's massive study of 120 cases. His opinion was that 'hystericals are, in general, not any more erotic than normal persons'. In *Principles of Psychotherapy* (1925), Janet promoted the view put forward by Christian Scientists, whose ideas he respected: 'a cure involved changing the influence that the sufferer's idea of his own troubles may have on the development of the disease. If the sufferer believes himself lost, the disease becomes so much the more serious; if he has confidence in his cure, the recovery is much more easy.'

Although Janet saw his patients' beliefs about their disease as central to their behaviour, he was not convinced that this was all there was to it:

> You could cure the sick by teaching them the truth about their disease. But what is the truth? Dubois tells them that they have no organic lesions. Dubois maintains that all the exhaustion of the psychasthenics depends simply on the 'idea of fatigue'.
>
> I am well aware that it is the fashion today to say that the hysteric is ill because she has taken it into her head to be ill, or because the physician has put the notion into her head. That is obviously very simple, but is it the whole truth? There are some who doubt it.

In 1901, Janet pointed out: 'The notion of psychotherapy is very vague; it is not easy to understand its meaning or judge its importance. Psychotherapy is not a treatment of the mind, but by the mind.'

In Vienna, Wilhelm Fleiss, an ear, nose and throat specialist with a considerable reputation as a healer, conducted surgery on the mucosa in the upper nasal passages of his patient, Emma Eckstein, in the belief it would cure her of masturbation and menstruation difficulties. Freud explored this approach before he made his abortive and disingenuous foray into a theory of the cause of hysteria in childhood seduction. This involved the attribution of what were then called hysterical symptoms to what would now be called child sexual abuse.

At this period of his career, Freud was still searching for the causes of his patients' experiences. His later theories and therapies were concerned with the meaning of the symptoms and he took note of conflicts and desires. Freud was aware that hysterical symptoms were imprecise recollections of past events when he commented that 'Hysterics suffer, mainly from reminiscences' (Breuer & Freud 1896).

At the time Freud was publishing in Vienna, physicians elsewhere were propounding other nervous theories. In the United States, George Beard (1880, 1881) popularised 'nervous exhaustion', 'neuraesthenia' and 'American nervousness'.

Hysteria grew into a standard diagnosis resulting in wider sections of the population being medicalised. Psychogenic theories retained their dominance through the twentieth century but, according to Shorter (1992), somatizing patients did not seek out psychiatrists.

Instead, they attended physicians and gynaecologists who had available legitimating diagnoses in terms of bodily diseases, and who were able to provide therapeutic interventions to match their formulations.

THE DISAPPEARANCES OF HYSTERIA

Within a decade of Charcot's death in 1893 and 20 years after the publication of Freud and Breuer's *Studies in Hysteria,* Charcot's pupils rejected the very diagnosis and the epidemic was said to be 'spent' (Appignanesi & Forrester 1992).

According to Janet (1925), physicians began to talk of the dangers of the treatments that they had recommended as being inoffensive and beneficial only a few years earlier. Furthermore, they began to make charges of immorality against the doctor for becoming involved in suggestion as a treatment. Their argument was that treatment by suggestion lowered the dignity of the physician and caused him to take on the attitude of a miracle worker.

In his extended study of this period, the first three decades of the twentieth century, Janet tried to find some explanation for the 'neglect and decay that had followed so closely on such enthusiasm and development'. At that time psychology was a confused mixture of literature and ethics, with no standing in the schools of medicine.

Armin Steyerthal, a director of a private health spa near Halle, wrote of hysteria, 'There is no such disease and has never been' (Micale 1994). The decline in acknowledging it continued and, in 1914, Paul Guiraud commented, in *Annales medico-psychologiques,* that, 'For some time now, one has no longer dared to speak of hysteria'. Hysteria disappeared, perhaps again into the consulting rooms of those who treated diseases of the uterus, of bones and joints, only to reappear on an unparalleled scale during World War I. Each war, since and before, has had its own distinct neurosis, and each has reflected the prevailing threats of its time.

In the 1960s, the standard British textbook, by Mayer-Gross, Slater and Roth, contained the following evidence of the profession's confusion:

In British psychiatry, it is common to call those states hysterical in which some motivation for symptoms can be discovered. The distinction of those states from malingering then becomes one of theoretical difficulty and needs the postulation of an 'unconscious' in which in the hysteric motivation remains submerged, or of some other hypothetical mechanism. In practice, the hysteric is not infrequently a malingerer too; and patients are seen whom all would call hysterical, where motivation remains speculative even after intensive inquiry.

Kirmayer and Robbins (1991) noted that somatizing patients did not like or easily accept psychological explanations. Shorter (1992) observed that doctors hated treating intangible symptoms. He believed that the great majority of emotionally caused illnesses could accurately be classified as purely psychogenic, hence somatoform. They were more likely to be classed as 'psychosomatic' simply because doctors preferred to intervene on behalf of their manifestations and not their causes.

Micale wrote about the second disappearance of hysteria. In 1994 he reported that a computer search of *Index Medicus* for the second half of the twentieth century produced titles such as *The End of Hysteria* and *Eclipse of Hysteria* and that, in a 1976 editorial, the *British Medical Journal* described hysterical neuroses as 'a virtual historical curiosity in Britain'. 'Where has all the hysteria gone?' asked an author in the *Psychoanalytic Review* in 1979. A few years later, a perplexed Jacques Lacan asked: 'Where are all the hysterics of former times, those magnificent women, the Anna Os and Emmy von Ns? What today has replaced the hysterical symptoms of Freud's time?' (*Economist* 4 May 1991).

The short answer is that some of Freud's women would have been re-diagnosed in the later twentieth century as personality-disordered and somatizing. As well, there has been a worldwide increase in both incidence and prevalence of medical procedures. In the absence of certainty of diagnosis, it could be that some of this increase is accounted for by doctors following the 'better safe than sorry' rule.

According to the account of John C. Nemiah published in the standard North American psychiatric textbook: 'It was often stated that conversion disorder was less frequently seen in psychiatric practice than it was 70 or 80 years ago' (Kaplan et al. 1980). According to Mace (1992), conversion hysteria was threatened with expulsion from classifications of psychiatric disorders, but criticism of its face validity had not led to adequate diagnostic alternatives.

The increase in medical remedies, surgical interventions and medicaments in use suggests that much of what was called hysteria is now attracting treatment under a disease label.

MODELS OF EXPLANATION FOR SERIOUS ILLNESS WITHOUT A DISEASE BASE

Edward Shorter (1992) points out that medicine has known that pain can arise in the mind since John Gregory wrote about it in 1770: 'Although the fears of these patients are generally groundless, their sufferings are real'.

In the 1930s, the word psychosomatic was coined, as many conditions not involving disease were recognised to be of psychological origin (Shorter 1985, 1992). Emotions such as anger and anxiety caused significant and measurable biochemical changes and affected the performance of internal organs. Emotions can bring about disease, especially if they are allowed to persist. For example, the increased secretion of stomach acid associated with repeated arousal to rage will bring about a peptic ulcer in an individual who is susceptible because he already has an infection. Symptom production in psychosomatic disorders is assumed to be mediated by the autonomic nervous system and through the release of hormones, leading to changes in heart rate, gut motility or stomach acid secretion. This 1930s description of psychosomatic disorders corresponded with changes caused in bodily functions without the person's thinking consciously about it. The body reacts before the mind is aware.

In 1980 somatization theory was introduced. It focused attention on the experience and expression of symptoms consequent on social factors. Excess symptom production in somatization is thought to be entirely psychogenic. The distribution of symptoms is determined in the mind, by ideas and beliefs, perhaps mapped out on the brain. Symptoms are referred onto body parts that have been sensitised by a variety of mechanisms, including earlier experiences of disease, the family history, prevalent epidemics and cultural beliefs. Somatization is thought to be the mechanism involved in the production of phantom pain. After trauma has necessitated amputation, the memory of pain and other sensations can be referred onto absent limbs that are experienced as if they are still in place.

The finding of both somatization phenomena and psychosomatic symptoms still does not exclude the possibility that there is co-existing disease. It is important to keep in mind that somatization might co-exist with, mask or actually be fostered by a disease, even one which does not have specific manifestations. It is mandatory to perform a thorough physical examination of every patient who is suspected of somatizing (Lipowski 1987a).

The category of 'psychological factors affecting physical condition' accommodates the notion that psychosocial stress can impinge on both the course and the experience of any disease. It is applied to clinical situations rather than to disease categories, encouraging physicians to think of the psychosomatic process as a dimension of a disease (Kirmayer & Robbins 1991; DSM-IIIR 1987). In 1984, Henker summed up the concept of psychosomatic medicine authoritatively: 'Practically any illness may be significantly influenced by mental processes'.

The concept of somatization involves a range of sensations, from uncomfortable to agonising, and accommodates indisposition and disability with no ascertainable cause (Shorter 1992). One hundred years after Freud, Merskey asserted that chronic pain was the most common manifestation of hysteria in the late twentieth century.

Szasz also suggests that most patients with hysteria are in the hands of doctors who fail to recognise it and treat it as if it were the disease it suggests or mimics.

PSYCHOSOMATIC ILLNESS AND SOMATIZATION

The symptoms of somatizing patients and their explanations have changed repeatedly over the last two centuries. According to Shorter (1992), the interpretations of patients tend to be chronologically ahead of those of the doctors who deal with them. This suggests that practising physicians learn how to treat patients from the media, popular literature, gossip and hearsay, and from patients themselves, not from medical or scientific sources. (Patients are now informed by the Internet and its tens of thousands of sites on RSI, all authoritatively placed, from Harvard to Tokyo.) In the case of the RSI epidemic, not only physicians but also scientific journals and institutions were dominated by laymen's views.

Explanations for hysterical symptoms ranged from 'irritation of the reflex arc', 'spinal irritation' and 'unstable colon' to 'reflexes from the sex organs' with the uterus as the leading player. Into the 1920s, neither lack of therapeutic success nor weakness of theoretical justification deterred reputable surgeons in England from removing the uterus as a treatment for hysteria.

With increasing awareness of its psychogenic origins, the term neurosis became psychoneurosis. The highly emotional person who complained of symptoms of organic disease but did not have clinical signs of such a disease was said to be suffering from hysteria, while the term neuraesthenia was revived to account for those presenting with nervous exhaustion and depression. The psychoneuroses became the province of psychotherapists, who focused their attention on the emotional matters that comprised their presumed aetiologies, not on the bodies in which they manifested.

In the 1950s psychoneurosis came to mean anxiety and depression and hysteria became an unfashionable term. The description 'neurotic' had re-emerged as an abbreviation, but it was removed from the American Psychiatric Association's diagnostic categories (DSM-III) in 1980, together with the term 'neurosis' and the similarly discredited 'neuraesthenia'. The residual somatic states, no longer the focus of attention, remained in a list of psychiatric diagnoses as hysterical neurosis or conversion symptoms, and these formed the basis of the broader concept of somatization, which was brought in and retained.

At the same time, where an emotional conflict manifested as a mental state suggestive of psychosis, the concept of hysteria was found underpinning a category of dissociative disorders, fugue states, multiple personality disorder, recovered memories, automatism, and borderline states sometimes manifesting as pseudologia fantastica, all of which spawned controversy about their nature. These were previously considered to be manifestations of hysterical personality disorder.

In common speech, the adjective 'hysterical' came to refer to overly emotional states. The caricatured personality of an immature, seductive but frigid female was termed 'hysterical' and was more recently accommodated within the framework of histrionic and borderline personality disorders. This pejorative view of hysteria, with its sexual overtones, made it an unpopular diagnosis, so nominal attributions for psychogenic symptoms came to be preferred by diagnosticians. The generally cited reason is that psychiatric diagnoses are stigmatising.

THE CHANGE TO THE SOMATOFORM DISORDERS

The medical world's views of disease are influenced by two diagnostic systems: the *International Classification of Diseases* of the World Health Organization (ICD) and the *Diagnostic and Statistical Manual* of the American Psychiatric Association (DSM), both appended with the number of the relevant edition.

Under pressure from feminist critics of psychiatry, the editors of the ICD-10 proposed not only that the name 'hysteria' be removed from its listing, but that reference to the concept of conversion should disappear as well. Unconscious motivation and secondary gain were not to be included in the guidelines or criteria for its diagnosis. An interim category, *conversion/dissociation disorder*, was proposed to assist with getting rid of hysteria entirely. This at least rectified the earlier split between (hysterical) conversion and (hysterical) dissociation and introduced a new category, *dissociative disorders of function and sensation*, and it acknowledged that their aetiologies were shared. ICD cautioned against making the diagnosis at all, suggesting that 'It now seems best to avoid the term "hysteria" as far as possible in view of its many and varied meanings'.

No caveats were issued, however, concerning the stigmatising effects of making an incorrect diagnosis, of treating non-existent conditions, or of placing people into a disease-based sick role. Paramedical professionals who used these diagnostic systems were no longer warned about the dangers of treating the mental content that was previously recognised as a dissociative phenomenon, confabulation, as if it were memory. Pointing out the consequences of making type II errors was left to historians and sociologists and did not become a concern for the medically qualified designers of diagnostic systems.

The American Psychiatric Association created the official taxonomy of agreed psychiatric knowledge to be used by psychiatrists, institutions and third-party payers. It was descriptive and resolutely atheoretical nosology, except when it came to somatization:

> The essential features of this group of disorders are physical symptoms suggesting physical disorder (hence somatoform) for which there are no demonstrable organic findings or known physiological mechanisms and for which there is positive evidence or a strong presumption that the symptoms are linked to psychological factors or conflicts.
>
> Although the symptoms of somatoform disorders are 'physical', the specific patho-physiological processes involved are not demonstrable or understandable by existing laboratory procedures and are conceptualised most clearly using psychological constructs.
>
> Symptom production is not under voluntary control: that is, the individual does not experience the sense of controlling their production.

Conversion disorder was unique in that underlying theory implied two specific mechanisms to account for the disturbance. In one, an individual achieves a primary gain by fulfilling a need or solving a conflict of desires while keeping it out of awareness. In the other, the individual achieves a secondary gain by avoiding an activity that is noxious or by getting support that otherwise might not be forthcoming (DSM-III 1980). But it warns that a symptom is not to be called hysterical when it is 'a culturally approved response to stress'.

Where legislation has been enacted in an injury model, RSI has become culturally approved at the highest level. Where no such approval exists, undiagnosable symptoms are seen as hysterical. This conundrum shows the self-serving arguments involved in maintaining hysteria as a psychiatric disorder. Either the number of psychiatric disorders needs to expand to accommodate all the cases, or a new language is needed to contain what it cannot explain when there is nothing at all wrong. History suggests that the expansionist tendencies of medicine and psychiatry are likely to prevail.

The underlying theory shows what might, or might not, be a rational intervention to which the symptoms could be expected to submit. Physical treatments cannot represent rational activity in alleviating the condition, as physical remedies are irrelevant to the resolution of the conflict or need which is at the base of the symptom. At the same time, such disease-focused remedies reinforce false beliefs about the body. One might further argue that their administration discourages attention to the real cause of the problem, the need or conflict combining with the belief and opportunity that the doctor provides.

Journals devoted to somatization carry advertisements for psychoactive drugs, which are fostering physical interventions. When somatization is a somatic manifestation of anxiety or depression, the underlying mood state of depression may submit to chemical intervention. When the symptom is a manifestation of a conflict or need, it will not respond. A physician might not countenance a physical treatment if somatization is clearly characterised as a process, governed by a set of beliefs and behaviour taking place in a context where it brings advantage.

Researchers in the United Kingdom and Canada have tried to understand the meaning of being sick (Lipowski 1968, 1986, 1987a, 1987b). One British group researched the relationship between life events and somatization in general practices in a region near London (Craig et al. 1994). Another group of British researchers stressed the universality of the phenomenon of somatization and its role as communication (Goldberg & Blackwell 1970; Goldberg & Bridges 1985; Goldberg, Bridges et al. 1987; Goldberg, Grayson et al. 1987). They are social psychiatrists and they conduct their research in general practice settings. They decline to claim jurisdiction over the area and they do not label the condition of somatizing subjects as psychiatric.

The British researchers deem somatization to be at the interface of medicine and psychiatry and they enlisted the participation of the primary care sector, where most of it is managed. They offer support, education and practical training for primary care practitioners in the use of techniques to manage somatizing patients. They encourage patients to re-attribute their symptoms to the stresses of everyday life rather than continue to think of themselves as suffering from an undiagnosed disease or from one not as yet understood (Goldberg 1992). This would assist them to care for themselves and have a beneficial effect on the utilisation of health services.

DEFINING SOMATIZATION

There has been no general agreement on a definition, not even on which elements amongst the behaviour, actions, beliefs, reasons, motives, desires or experiences of somatizing patients should be the focus of medical interest. Different observers, from different vantage points, interpret somatization as having different meanings. Psychiatrists, especially those working in developing countries, agree on this if nothing else: from Bahrain to Borneo, the most common way that emotional distress and psychiatric illness to present is in the form of somatic symptoms (Murphy 1989).

The first use of the term is attributed to Stekel, as an equivalent of conversion (Stekel 1943). The second edition of *Gould's Medical Dictionary* (1956) identifies somatization with conversion but distinguishes it from psychosomatic disorder: 'a psychoneurotic displacement of emotional conflicts onto muscles and sensory apparatus innervated by the voluntary nervous system, in distinction to psychosomatic reaction in which displacement occurs onto organs and viscera innervated by the autonomic system'.

Lipowski (1968) saw somatizing patients as a psychologically and psychiatrically heterogenous group and he focused on somatic metaphors as communication through which the patients seek medical help. Lipowski adopted a purely descriptive definition to accommodate the difficulty of verifying, in universally acceptable research terms, what he suspected (but could not prove) to be the causal role of accompanying psychosocial distress. Kirmayer pointed out that somatization is properly viewed as a variant of illness behaviour and help-seeking and that the relationship between somatization and psychiatric disorder is an empirical question rather than a definitional one (Kirmayer & Robbins 1991).

Katon, Ries and Kleinman (1984) focused on symptoms as communication and defined somatization as 'an idiom of distress in which patients with psychosocial and emotional problems articulate their distress, primarily through physical symptomatology'.

The Kleinmans researched cross-cultural psychiatry, finding somatic presentations of distress to be the norm rather than the exception (Kleinman & Kleinman 1985). They defined somatization as 'an expression of personal and social distress in an idiom of bodily complaints with medical help seeking'. Their patients attended a psychiatric clinic in Hunan, a province of China, and their overview incorporated the role of the physician. In this transactional view of somatization, doctors sanction the patients' bodily idiom of distress. In the view of Arthur Kleinman (1988):

> The concept of somatization is predicated on the belief that psychological and biological vulnerability combine with local social pressures to create syndromes of distress embodying neuroendocrine, autonomic, cardiovascular, gastrointestinal and limbic system responses and that such responses constitute a spectrum of affective, anxiety and somatic complaints.

This definition accommodates psychosomatic responses, the best known of which is the increase in heart rate that results from getting a fright. Somatoform and psychosomatic responses cannot be separated in practice, particularly in an anxious patient.

Because somatization goes back several centuries and is worldwide in its distribution, Goldberg and Bridges suggested that perhaps it should be regarded as a basic human mechanism for responding to stress: we develop pains and discomfort in our bodies. They pointed out that recourse to the articulation of emotional problems in psychological terms is the more recent phenomenon, more common in richer developed countries, and to be expected in egocentric cultures where there is a narcissistic idealisation of the self. Somatization, on the other hand, is said to occur where the individual is submerged in a group.

Goldberg and Bridges (1985) note the adaptive advantages of somatization, painful though it might be in other ways. Somatizing allows the psychologically unwell to occupy the sick role without stigmatisation and to avoid responsibility for their lives and predicaments. Somatization is blame-avoiding. It is enough to be in pain; because one is hurting, one is eligible for the secondary gains of the sick role. Somatization saves patients from being as depressed or anxious as they might otherwise have been, given their predicaments.

The compensatory disadvantage seems to be that somatization lasts longer than a purely psychological disorder might in the same circumstances. Huxley and Goldberg (1975) take the view that it is the failure to face up to one's problems by changing attribution which is responsible for the greater tendency for the disorder to become chronic. Once somatization is established, it is easy to see how it continues. It secures advantages from the spouse, family and employers and tends to be encouraged by medical personnel. At the same time, doctors devalue emotional difficulties and predicaments for which there are no easy, in the sense of medical, solutions (Lipowski 1987b).

According to Murphy (1989), somatization currently refers to how patients seek medical help for bodily symptoms but incorrectly attribute them to organic disease.

In the United States, Charles Ford (1982) sidestepped the influence of dominant views and provided a definition of somatization better suited to sociological analysis. His view is that somatization is not a diagnosis, but a process 'by which the body, the soma, is used for psychological purposes or for personal gain'. By focusing on the apparent purpose of somatizing and seeking medical care, Ford incorporates the activity undertaken by doctors on behalf of somatization and he claims that it forms a large and lucrative industry.

Ford suspects that illness does not occur in the population in a normal distribution but that relatively few persons experience a disproportionately large number of illnesses. Either such persons are unusually prone to disease processes, or this group consists of persons who repetitively somatize. Because services of physicians are offered within a disease model, it is not unreasonable to propose that the treatment that somatizing patients receive is not very effective.

Ford believes that attention to the doctor–patient relationship would be a cost-effective enterprise, one that would help to ameliorate growing dissatisfaction with the technical virtuosity of medicine. He laments that physicians seem hesitant to change the manner in which they practise medicine.

Ford's definition emphasises the connection between getting sick and the benefits of the sick role. This is more sociological in thrust as, unlike psychiatric or psychologistic theories, it does not take the 'unconsciousness' of a subject's motivation for granted. Ford's broader perspective on somatization accommodates consciously motivated behaviours such as the Munchausen syndrome, a factitious disorder which presents with fabricated or tricked-up symptoms, knowingly feigned, put on to attract pity as well as investigations and procedures in a medical setting (Asher 1951). Only persons who somatize as a lifestyle are to be thought of as having somatoform disorders.

Ford adverts not only to the feelings in the body, but also to the action that the subjects take on their behalf. He declines to differentiate conscious from unconscious motivation towards illness. No diagnostician can read individual subjects' minds to know how aware they are of why they are really seeing the doctor. Somatizing patients repeatedly dismiss reassurance from trusted doctors and persistently seek out medical opinion to confirm their perceptions. In the setting of compensation, they select the most sympathetic physicians who are least likely to get them back to work. They are mindful of the consequences of their actions, but deny that they are motivated by them.

Ford goes on to list psychological gains to be made from somatization: the experience of unpleasant emotions as physical symptoms and alleviation of guilt. Personal gains flow from the capacity to manipulate interpersonal relationships: release from duties and responsibilities, absence from work, excuses not to complete housework, financial gain and entitlement to seek a closer relationship with and sympathy from another person.

THE MORAL ASPECTS OF DEALING WITH SOMATIZATION

As described by Ford, somatization accommodates two elements: first, the production of symptoms, which is involuntary, and, second, the action taken on their behalf, which is more knowingly sought out and settled on. The morally laden element is not that one experiences symptoms, as these are universal phenomena, but that one claims exemptions on their behalf. The physician in practice finds it difficult to separate the patient's feeling sick from what he should do about it.

The likelihood that a doctor will write a certificate is increased when that doctor's income depends on his patient's goodwill. He can use his power as the unquestioned expert; he is entitled to be angry if his certificate is not accepted. The doctor's advice removes a taint of moral infirmity from the patient as the doctor takes responsibility for his patient's moral dereliction.

A conscientious physician can invoke a dimension of sickness to assess if exemption is justifiable. It is possible to get an acceptable level of observer agreement as to whether a patient is sick or simply wants a certificate. Is he bedridden, crippled or impaired for day-to-day living? What does he do outside of the consulting room? Examination of the domestic and social exploits of somatizing patients reveals a full spectrum from invalidity to a manifest social advantage. The daring diagnostician might be tempted to believe that malingering can be distinguished from somatization. The gate-keeper might consider granting entitlement to exemptions on the basis of global dysfunction rather than the report of symptoms.

A person does not seem to have a choice in deciding if his or her depression, anxiety, or conflict will be expressed in a somatic mode where it must be suffered, or expressed in a psychological way so that it can be talked about. In some cultures, the presentation of mental disorder is entirely somatic. To whom and how a person presents his or her problems is a function of the culture, of legal arrangements and of the availability of intervention for one mode of presentation over the other. This is, in general terms, culture.

Not all somatizing subjects want to be in the sick role. Some remain preoccupied with bodily sensations while going about their business. The moral position of the physician is crucial to what happens. It dictates his response to a patient who is anxious, dependent, uninformed and willing to undertake any prescribed remedy. Will the physician take masterful but unsuccessful action? Will he administer a remedy for something to do? Will he feign confidence in physical remedies for transitory gain? Or will he be able to muster the tact and the restraint to understand a somatizing patient, for whose predicament there is no medical remedy?

Illich made the point that pain can mean suffering, sickness, illness, hunger, mourning or oppression. In 1974, Illich claimed that an increasing portion of pain was man-made and a side effect of strategies for industrial expansion. He argued that the medicalisation of pain served the interests of the physician who defined as medical the consequences of problems that he or she was unable to influence. Pain experienced in the body is the only part of human suffering over which the medical profession can claim competence and control. By adopting a medical stance, the physician accepted the sufferer as a patient and then he distilled a painful somatic state out of more diffuse suffering, priming that person to be treated by medical remedies.

Illich made the point that medical civilisation tends to turn pain and suffering into a technical matter, thereby depriving suffering of its inherent personal meaning and turning it into demands made by individuals on the economy, 'problems which can be managed or *produced* [his italics] out of existence. Culture makes pain tolerable by interpreting its necessity; only pain perceived as curable is intolerable.'

Morris, a cultural theorist, sees chronic pain in much the same way as Illich, as an immense, invisible crisis at the centre of contemporary life. He believes that Western medicine leads to misinterpretation of pain as no more than a sensation, a symptom and a problem in biochemistry. The failure of this traditional reading of pain creates and sustains this crisis. By taking back responsibility for how we understand pain we can recover the power to alleviate it (Morris 1991).

DID HYSTERIA REALLY DISAPPEAR?

This all suggests that hysteria did not disappear at all. Epidemic hysteria became subsumed in the literature of moral panics. The clinical entity of hysteria split in three directions: into the somatoform disorders, into new fashionable diseases managed by fringe practitioners and into conditions presented to clinicians who did not make a distinction between a physical condition and its psychogenic mimic. (Stewart 1990).

As drugs and exploratory procedures became safer, it became less important for a clinician to make the right diagnosis before intervening. The evidence suggests that much of what was formerly diagnosed as hysteria now passes for and is treated as organic disease.

The story of the development of the concept of somatization is the story of medicine's struggle with finding words to accommodate the notion of illness without disease and to keep it within its jurisdiction. Before its medicalisation, ill health was not a value-free issue. The quest to medicalise it was dogged, or perhaps propelled, by poorly articulated concerns about blame, virtue, character and motivation.

Underlying the enterprise is the medical profession's unending tendency to create a clientele and to understand the meaning of symptoms suspected of having a rationality of their own.

The category of somatization is indispensable to defeat those critics who suggested that illness was a moral issue and not entirely a medical one. If illness were a moral issue, it would not be the legitimate concern of doctors but of some priestly or quasi-bureaucratic caste of ethicists and moralists.

Illness not accounted for by disease became somatization.

The notion of somatization adverts only to the agenda of patients. The medical profession might have to take responsibility for the role of the physician in fostering it. From the indifferent viewpoint of the social theorist, diseased people, malingerers and somatizers can all be seen as motivated to adopt the sick role and to capitalise on its benefits.

From the viewpoint of society, there is a crucial distinction between somatization and faking it. This is a moral one, invoked only if the subject is found to be telling lies. A worthwhile enterprise for a health-policy economist would be an analysis of the physician's role in the suggestion and reinforcement of symptoms.

From the viewpoint of a psychiatrist, the patient's motivation towards illness might be of concern, but one does not need an expert to know that.

From the viewpoint of the forensic psychiatrist giving evidence in court cases, the nub of the matter is that somatoform symptoms are caused by mental events, beliefs, emotions and predicaments, and not by physical trauma. The judge is, or should be, concerned with their causes.

With these conceptual tools, illness, disease, somatization, needs, desires, reasons, motives and predicaments, we can now move to the case in question, a set of somatoform symptoms known as writers' cramp.

All clinical descriptions of cramp fulfil the criteria for a diagnosis of somatization, so a review of the literature on writers' cramp and some earlier epidemics may elucidate some characteristics of the social milieu in which this particular symptom complex became epidemic before and how it produced occupational impairment on a scale that caused medical, legal, economic and social concern.

3

PERCEPTIONS OF WRITERS' CRAMP AND ITS EPIDEMICS

Of course, so long as patients do not write,
they are a great deal more comfortable than when
they write much, or make futile attempts to do so.
But how many return to their desk after a holiday ...
only to find, to their grievous disappointment,
that the rebellion of the hand against the mind
continues just as strong as before, or that, if it did
appear suppressed for a few days, it was suppression
like that of the Cuban insurrection, which subsequent
mail shows to be undaunted, in spite of ministerial
announcements and parliamentary misgivings.

Julius Althaus, Physician, 1870

Writers' cramp is the common name for motor and sensory symptoms that interfere with the performance of a manual task, or a disturbance of function and sensation in upper limbs that suggests illness or injury. Cramp can occur without local pathology, as a functional disorder, or secondary to local disease as functional overlay. The controversy about its nature has not reached closure, but treatable organic causes are improbable.

Literally hundreds of specific occupational cramps, some of them archaic, have been named in many languages, as well as more generic craft neurosis, fatigue disease, functional spasm, occupational neurosis, professional impotence, professional hyperkinesis, and steel nib and scriveners' palsy.

Accounts of cramp all describe a plethora of clinical manifestations, provide endless suggestions concerning morbid anatomy and refer to concurrent emotional symptomatology. X-rays, muscle biopsies, nerve conduction studies, computerised axial tomography scans, magnetic resonance imaging and positron emission tomography have not added to knowledge of the disorder. Its psychic determinants remain unexamined and no-one has charted its natural history. The controversy about its nature has not reached closure. Treatable peripheral lesions appear improbable.

Transient cramp is a familiar sensation, but the literature concerns an enduring affliction. Writers' cramp has never been definitively classified. Attempts include 'motor and sensory'; 'spasmodic and paralytic' (Gowers 1888); 'tremulous and neuralgic' (Jelliffe 1910); 'primary and true' (Head 1910); 'spasm, manipulation difficulties and symptoms' (Great Britain and Ireland Post Office 1911); 'tremulous, spastic, ataxic or physiogenic' (Pai 1947); 'painful and non-painful' and 'simple, progressive and dystonic' (Sheehy & Marsden 1982). Every case is different, even within the same occupational category. All types merge with one another and change in the course of the affliction.

Cramp was first recognised by Ramazzini in *De Morbis Artificum (The Diseases of Workers)* (1700). He identified tension, local tiredness, constant sitting and constant strain on the mind as causes of maladies among scribes.

1830s: THE ENGLISH CIVIL SERVICE AND THE STEEL NIB

The first epidemics of writers' cramp were reported in the 1830s among male clerks of the English Civil Service, who attributed it to a new technology, the steel nib (Bell 1833). Sir Charles Bell described cramp under the caption of *Partial Paralyses of the Muscles of the Extremities* and was the first to comment on a relationship between the conflicted will and the symptom (Bell 1854). He wrote: 'The nerves and muscles are capable of their proper functions and proper adjustments; the defect is in the imperfect exercise of the will, or in the secondary influence the brain has over the relations established in the body'.

Tenosynovitis was first proposed to be the cause of writers' cramp in 1840 by Georg Freidrich Strohemeyer, whose unsuccessful surgical approach of cutting and separating tendons was dismissed quickly as overzealous, naive and unsuccessful. William Osler, the Canadian physician, reported that Strohemeyer 'opened the way to the folly of surgical treatment by tenotomy, which still prevails in many of the analogous conditions such as tics and wry neck' (1910).

In 1864 Samuel Solly, a surgeon, reported on 'scriveners' palsy' and that 'the greatest part of the middle classes of London got their bread by the use of the pen recording the sums lost, or spent in this vast Babylon'. Solly treated his patients with rest, strychnine and firm reassurance. His case histories acknowledge the role of fatigue and emotional factors. He warned:

> Upon your early correct diagnosis may depend the health and happiness of your subject. If you mistake its real nature and regard it as a sign of incipient softening of the brain, a mistake I have known to occur, you may destroy the happiness of your patient and bring on the very disease which you have erroneously diagnosed.

Sir John Russell Reynolds rejected the view that cramp was caused by excessive exertion, because thousands of individuals worked without suffering. He observed worry and anxiety in cramp subjects and noted that he had seen a case in a person who had been very interested in the occurrence of symptoms in a friend. He reasoned that, if a motor nerve were damaged a muscle would be palsied, and if a sensory nerve were damaged then sensation would be defective. Reynolds understood the role of the will and in 1878 published a paper called *Disturbances of Function and Sensation Dependent on Idea*.

1872: POORE IN GREAT BRITAIN

In 1872 George Vivian Poore, an authority on sanitation, jurisprudence and medical uses of electricity, published a report of a single case of writers' cramp.

His patient, George Gair, a 32-year-old clerk in excellent health, intelligent and well educated, was engaged in nine hours of writing a day. His symptoms had started suddenly when he described difficulty in bringing his hand down on the paper. He tried unsuccessfully to hold his right hand down with his left and eventually had to leave his employment. Gair learnt to write with his left hand, but that became involved as well.

Poore noted that there was only a perversion of function, motor symptoms being prominent rather than the more commonly reported sensory ones. When Gair undressed, twitches were evident in his pectoral muscles, his arm was tense in various muscle groups at various times and his thumb and fingers went into spasm with any allusion to them.

In spite of these difficulties, Gair attempted treatments including manual labour, digging, sea bathing in cold water, exercises with dumbbells, rowing and gymnastics, all with no benefit. A sea voyage was prescribed, so Gair worked as a steward, but his specific disability showed no improvement. Poore recommended galvanism twice a week, Pulvermacher's chain bands (which caused scars), cold shower baths, and friction with horsehair gloves every morning. The spine was to be rubbed with croton oil three or four times a week, as well as creams and various oils supplemented by small doses of strychnine. Rest was ineffective, so total rest in a plaster cast was prescribed; with that, the spasms became worse.

Poore reasoned that if a stammerer could often sing, then normal rhythmical movement would assist his patient to return to writing. He employed electric batteries rhythmically to stimulate the arm. He added a quarter of a grain of morphia a day and Gair's improvement was sudden and remarkable. Instead of returning to his former occupation, the patient was able to start a small business.

Poore believed that he had treated Gair by the joint use of galvanic current and exercise. The record showed that successful treatment had involved listening to a detailed life story, administering a powerful sedative, morphia, and re-educating him in rhythm and relaxation. We would now call this combination sedation, analgesia, taking an interest and relaxation therapy.

His success brought Poore a great number of referrals and in December 1878 he published *An Analysis of 75 Cases of Writers' Cramp and Impaired Writing Power.* Poore charted all the muscles that seemed to be involved and reasoned that all the upper torso muscles were used in writing, so all of them could have been affected.

Poore reported that there was an emotional factor in every case but he still adhered to his notion of central changes in the face of a variety of symptoms. Initially he believed that there was a writing centre somewhere in the brain and that it was being stimulated into disharmony by the act of writing. He submitted that the crossover of symptoms to the unused arm could be explained by an analogy to the inflammation, as if in sympathy, of one eye following a traumatic injury to the other. This is called 'sympathetic ophthalmoplegia.'

Poore did not suggest that an excess of writing had been the cause, as some of his patients had not done much writing at all — one had developed cramp after a single day's work.

When some of Poore's patients reported that their symptoms extended to lower limbs, the phenomenon could no longer be attributed to a task-precipitated local origin. Poore then postulated a different and local cause for each manifestation. He did not report again on his patients' emotional difficulties, nor on their social problems. He persisted with his panaceas and reported no more successes.

Poore's classification of cramp was an example of symptom diagnosis, based on description. Rather than differentiate the organic from the functional cases, he attributed a hypothetical organicity to them all. Where the predominant symptom was pain, he called it 'neuritic' or 'neuralgic'. He saw the pain as originating in peripheral nerves, whereas the motor symptoms originated in the brain, perhaps in a 'writing centre'. Only the dystonic cases, those in which muscle tone was abnormal, were to be regarded as 'true' writers' cramp.

1879: BEARD IN THE UNITED STATES

As interest in treatment of the formerly rare condition grew, an American study, *Conclusions from the Study of 125 Cases of Writer's Cramp and Allied Affections* (Beard 1879) was published in *The Medical Record*. Beard drew his generalisations from the variety of symptoms rather than characteristics of patients.

George Beard was a pioneer neurologist who made his reputation treating the functional nervous disorders, for which no gross pathology could be found. He was best known for his popularisation of neurasthenia, which he insisted was 'a real disease' (Beard 1880; Sicherman 1977). Because neurological disorders were rarely treatable, specialists welcomed patients with less tangible ills. Beard had an unshakeable belief in organic causes and he retained an unwarranted faith in his capacity to cure them with the nostrums of the period. He was an entrepreneur. He never questioned his licence to subject his willing patients to empirical remedies.

Although he considered writers' cramp to be a misnomer, Beard suggested that to substitute another term would heighten the confusion in the face of imperfect and changing knowledge of its pathology. He concluded that the disease was 'both peripheral and central' and that it might affect any point between the periphery and the centre. He agreed with Poore that there was a writing centre but, by the time Beard wrote about it in America, Poore, in London, had changed his mind and dismissed the idea.

Beard believed that cramp was a disease of the strong and that it was more easily cured in the strong. He also believed that it was a disease less likely to attack those who did original work, such as authors and journalists, than clerks who did routine work. He attributed this to the fact that original workers had to stop to think. He reported a case of cramp in an authoress who had performed a single task of copying one afternoon. By conferring with physicians who saw it only rarely, Beard confirmed that there was a regional variation in its prevalence, with southern states less affected than the northern.

Beard suggested numerous remedies: electric and galvanic therapies, massage, friction, pinching and pounding of the skin, passive movements of the joints, dry heat, dry cold, hot water and ice, cautery and producing small blisters along the course of what he believed to be 'affected nerves and muscles'. He prescribed doses of castor oil, iodides, fats and tonics. He advocated penholders, quills and pens with broad nibs, using a lead pencil, writing with the left hand, typewriting, rowing and paddling. He noted that turning doorknobs and carrying bundles hurt some subjects but not others.

1886: LEWIS IN THE UNITED STATES

In 1886 an American, Dr Morris Lewis, attempted the most substantial literature review of cramp that had been done to that time. Part of the charm of this 40-page report with 120 references lies in its documentation of all the remedies that reappeared in the therapeutic armamentaria of clinicians a century later. Tenotomy alone was reported as unsuccessful. Lewis named the muscles, nerves, spinal and other tissues that various authorities thought to be been involved. He reported on popular theories and hypotheses concerning pathology or morbid anatomy. Duchenne, Solly, Reynolds, Althaus, Brown-Séquard, Romberg all advocated purely central pathology. Weir Mitchell attributed the involvement of the unused hand to 'hyper sensitising of the sensory centre'.

Every empirical remedy that had ever been mentioned was documented by Lewis as being in use, as well as nerve stretching, administering a blow to the neck, various mechanical appliances, rings which held the pen attached to the wrist by rubber bands, penholders, Velpeau's apparatus of an oval ball of hard rubber around the pen, a board moving on rollers to put under the hand, and subcutaneous atropine. Each remedy was recommended to match a local symptom that needed to be relieved. There was no attempt to distinguish the management of cramps that had an organic basis from those that did not. Psychogenesis did not enter Lewis's repertoire, nor did his case histories advert to personal matters.

1888: GOWERS AND THE SHIFT TO OCCUPATIONAL NEUROSIS

William Gowers was the leading English neurologist at a time when neurology was a most advanced area in British medicine. Writers' cramp had again progressed from being a rare disease to a common one. By 1888 cramp had been reported in more than 80 occupations, most of which did not involve either rapid movements or repetitive work. Gowers reported cramp in typists as soon as typewriters were introduced. While Poore had conceptualised writers' cramp as a disorder caused by the antecedent task, Gowers invoked the German term 'occupation neurosis'. In this way, he effected a shift from a theory of physical causation in peripheral tissues to the idea of functional nervous disorder with symptoms excited by the act of writing. He suspected a hereditary tendency and noted the subjects' susceptibility to anxiety.

Gowers understood that the pain was referred to muscles, bones and joints or to the position of certain nerves, suggesting neuralgia, from which cramp differed in being excited rather than caused by a specific action. He distinguished 'motor and sensory' and 'spasmodic and neuralgic' forms but noted that, in practice, these were all combined. In describing the characteristics of over 100 cases, he noted that cramp was a 'disease easily imagined by those who have witnessed the disorder'. Subjects had a 'distinctly nervous' temperament and were 'irritable, sensitive and bearing overwork and anxiety badly'. Gowers remarked on 'the number of sufferers enduring anxiety from family trouble, business worry or weighty responsibilities'. Cramp occasionally followed local disease, injury or ill health and Gowers reported on his difficulties in differentiating a genuine case from a feigned one, a problem that continues to challenge the courts and medical examiners of today.

When Gowers reported on symptoms that spread to the unused arm he attributed this phenomenon to an origin in the central nervous system. To Gowers, 'true cramp' was only the dystonic, or spastic, variety. He considered vague pains and discomforts to be 'imagined cramp', resulting from fear of developing it, a state of affairs for which he recommended firm reassurance, apparently with some success. Unlike Lewis, who declared all remedies to be successful, Gowers reported the failure of the whole range, including Indian hemp. He found re-education in writing style to be helpful and advocated a relaxed hand with sweeping strokes and rhythmic movements.

Gowers understood the role of temperament, of domestic stress causing anxiety, and probably of other emotional factors. He understood the role of both suggestion and suggestibility but he did not comment on the role of popular beliefs. In today's terminology, Gowers would be a behaviour therapist who was aware of his patients' psychosocial difficulties.

Gowers located cramp among the neuroses, related it to personal and emotional factors and made available a reasonably effective remedy in the form of education and attention to predicament. These changes in the management of cramp might have been factors in decreasing its capacity to disable, at least at the hands of physicians who followed his ideas.

There was no retrievable literature on cramp for the next 20 years.

1907–11: TELEGRAPHISTS' CRAMP

In 1907 telegraphists' cramp was added to the Third Schedule of diseases covered by the British Workman's Compensation Act (1906), on the evidence of the union's physician, Dr Sinclair, who testified that cramp was 'muscular failure, caused by the rapid repetitive movements of telegraphy' and that three per cent of telegraphists suffered from it. The Postal Telegraphist Clerks Association wanted changes in their industrial arrangements and used the fact that Dr Sinclair had defined various aspects of their working conditions as its causes. As a consequence of Sinclair's lobbying, Morse telegraphy came to be included in the growing list of dangerous trades, along with writing. The scheduling of telegraphists' cramp reflected the capacity of a strategic service to exert pressure on government. An epidemic of cramp followed the decision to make it a compensable disorder.

The medical profession was again confused and numerous theories of causation were proposed. Some thought it was an inflammation of tendons, but it was rarely localised and, unlike tenosynovitis, it neither resolved nor led to stenosis. Some thought cramp to be a disease of peripheral nerve entrapments, but agreement could not be reached as to whether nerves had been compromised at the wrist, the elbow, the brachial plexus or as they left the spinal column. Medical and surgical interventions abounded, yet the increasing prevalence of cramp stood testimony to the physicians' lack of success. Sensory symptoms of various kinds were reported and these involved the unused arm and even the legs and back, contradicting any theory of local task-related origin. Such physical theories of causation as existed could not be linked to the occupational tasks, nor could they accommodate the emerging epidemiology of the disorder.

In 1911, the Great Britain and Ireland Departmental Committee into Telegraphists' Cramp was called '... to inquire into the prevalence and causes of the disease known as telegraphists' cramp and to report what means might be adopted for its prevention'.

The inquiry was held against the push for both improved working conditions and job security for Morse telegraphists. The Committee created three categories to account for reports: 'symptoms', 'difficulties in manipulation' and 'spasm'. Echoing Gowers, it suggested that some people had 'imagined cramp.' The Committee defined 'true cramp' as only the dystonic form, that with visible spasm. Up to 60 per cent of the workforce in one section were reporting 'symptoms', 30 per cent were experiencing 'difficulties in manipulation' and three per cent had 'spasmodic cramp'. The overall proportion of telegraphists affected was 18 per cent. Males outnumbered females and the Committee attributed this 'to the fact that a large proportion of female telegraphists left the service after a much shorter period for marriage and other reasons'.

Inquiries undertaken concurrently in a number of European countries found only sporadic cases. Similar studies among the staff of the two major telegraphic firms in the United States revealed a four and ten per cent incidence of reporting 'symptoms' in the Western Union and the Postal Company, respectively, and found that US telegraphists had workloads three times those of British workers. In the United States, cramp was known as 'losing your grip' and was attributed to 'predisposition'.

In its first written submission provided to the inquiry, the Postal Telegraph Clerks Association listed the causes to which cramp was being attributed. These included constitutional weakness, inaptitude for telegraph work, the nature and amount of a telegraphist's work, the conditions under which it was done, a bad style of manipulation, too early responsibility, heavy manual work, the construction of

Morse keys, and inadequate working accommodation. However, studies of cases and conditions failed to support a correlation between the incidence of cramp and any of its imputed causes.

The Association then shifted ground and submitted that cramp was due to excessive workload. However, the opposite turned out to be the case, with the fastest night-shift news telegraphists, working for bonuses, not providing a single case. As the cases came under examination, the Postal Telegraph Clerks' Association gave up the discredited theories and proposed stress to be the cause of cramp. The relationship of stress to the development of cramp remained unexamined.

The Committee included three eminent physicians and reviewed the medical profession's ideas about what caused cramp, which included nerve entrapment, tendonitis, inflammation and muscular failure. The Committee concluded, on clinical grounds, against all of them. The conclusion was that cramp was a neurosis: 'the result of a weakening or breakdown in the central controlling mechanism of the brain, resulting in spasm and inco-ordination of muscles which perform the specific act of telegraphy'. The report continued: '...the nervous breakdown known as Telegraphists' Cramp is due to a combination of two factors, one, a nervous instability on the part of the operator and the other, repeated fatigue during the complicated movements required for sending messages'.

As the work was common to all telegraphic workers, yet not all developed cramp, the Committee concluded that 'the amount of fatigue required to cause cramp is governed solely by a personal factor and has no constant relation to the amount of work performed'. After extensive studies, it recommended: 'If the conditions that lead to fatigue ... can be remedied, the personal factor alone remains as a cause of cramp and this can only be eliminated by careful and judicious selection of staff'.

A 'neurasthenic temperament' was said to be a predisposing factor and subjects were described as 'nervous'. Some people were considered to be 'unsuitable' for telegraphist work as 'a neurasthenic telegraphist might believe those difficulties to be real as existed only in his imagination' and, occasionally, a telegraphist who wished to give up operative work might feign the symptoms of cramp.

Although it denied that the Association's attributions were in any way the causes of cramp, the Committee created a document advocating industrial standards to be maintained in regard to employment, training, accommodation, furniture, equipment, workloads and conditions, granting the Association all it desired. Industrial relationships had been successfully negotiated through a health agenda.

Writing and typing are still classified as dangerous trades in the United Kingdom and guidelines to the diagnosis of writers' cramp are published at regular intervals. These stipulate that only the painful, dystonic type, with visible spasm, is to be compensable as a prescribed disease and it is now known as prescribed disease A4 (PDA4).

1926: INDUSTRIAL FATIGUE RESEARCH BOARD

The inquiry into telegraphists' cramp spawned two streams of research, one into the effects of repetitive work and the other into the possibility of early identification of personal susceptibility to cramp (Burnett 1926; Smith et al. 1927). In the United Kingdom the Industrial Fatigue Board was approached by the Union of Post Office Workers in 1922 to investigate means of preventing the liability to telegraphists' cramp. Two distinct groups, those suffering from cramp and those apparently free of it, were studied intensively. Cramp subjects had a far greater susceptibility to muscular fatigue, less control when sending a message and less ability to perform quick and accurate movements, which confirmed their impaired capability.

Seventy-five per cent of cramp subjects and 32 per cent of the non-cramp controls attracted the diagnosis of a 'minor mental disturbance, a psycho-neurosis, characterised by anxiety, obsessions or hysteria', and this represented a twofold higher incidence of psychoneurotic symptoms among cramp subjects than among unaffected workers. The two groups were not completely differentiated by any of the tests, so there was no assurance that the propensity to develop cramp could be detected with certainty. One-third of the unaffected control subjects and three-quarters of those who were affected possessed predisposing characteristics for cramp, but only a small number of those who did not have cramp ever developed the condition. Procedures based on excluding psychoneurotic or anxious individuals were unacceptable as they would have excluded too many people who would never develop cramp.

No study of the social predicament of cramp subjects was undertaken, nor were the causes of their anxiety investigated.

Highly intelligent individuals were found to be unsuitable for repetitive work and a recommendation was made that they should be identified before they embarked on the wrong career. The individual determined the experience of monotony, not the work (Burnett 1926).

By 1926 there was diminishing work for Morse telegraphists, except in the armed forces, as the telephone, telex and wireless became preferred modes of communication.

1892–1920:
OSLER'S *PRINCIPLES AND PRACTICE* *OF MEDICINE*

Dr William Osler, while editing his own textbook, was careful not to assume a causal connection between an activity and the neurosis that occasionally followed it. He advised prophylactic measures based on a proper method of writing. Rest was to be an essential component of treatment and it was accompanied by attention to nutrition. He reported a case of writers' cramp in a gynaecologist but did not say if his patient was able to continue at work.

In 1910 William Osler and Thomas McCrae undertook a critical review of the literature of cramp, in which they divorced the symptom from the preceding occupation. They pointed out that the laryngologist would otherwise see preachers', singers' and auctioneers' cramps, the practitioner in rural districts would see milkers' palsies and the medical man in a miners' camp would treat pick cramp and miners' nystagmus. The increasing incidence of cramp in women was noted as they took over telegraphy, stenography and typewriting and engaged in manufacturing industry. Osler and McCrae's findings were consistent with cramp having mental causes: 'The multiplicity of forms described ... all arise on this common mental basis; they may be found isolated in one patient, or may exist in various combinations. All distinctions are arbitrary.' Forcing the patient to write with the other hand frequently resulted in double cramp.

After Osler's death in 1919, McCrae took over editing the textbook that still bore Osler's name. Although the section on occupational neuroses was still attributed to Osler, its text represented a regression to recommending old, empirical placebo remedies, which benefited doctors, not patients. Treatment was once again to proceed in a discredited physical modality, galvanic electricity. The historian of medicine might find it hard to attribute that shift to Osler himself.

1922–73:
PRICE'S *TEXTBOOK OF THE PRACTICE OF MEDICINE*

Collier and Adie wrote about cramp in sequential editions of Price's *Textbook of the Practice of Medicine* (1922–35) and saw the craft palsies as determined by the habitual use of one set of muscles. Their aetiology was central. Breakdown in function was located in the basal ganglia. Cramp was thought to be especially common in demobilised soldiers, who were included with cigar makers, cigarette rollers and gold beaters in the list of occupations known to be involved. Typing and telegraphy were classed as dangerous trades, but parliament ignored the distribution of cramp across the working population. Collier and Adie pointed out that 'the gold beater had to bear the brunt of his own incapacity'.

Collier and Adie later revived the notion that certain Morse instruments, but not others, should be abandoned because they produced cramp (Collier & Adie 1937). They reverted to seeing occupational causes but made no attempt to connect their hypothetical problem in the brain with a prior occupation. Good treatment was to consist of removal of adverse factors in the patients' working environment. These included uncomfortable conditions, poor light, excessive noise and sources of personal friction. Collier was emphatic that neurosis did not enter the picture. Nonetheless, he recommended psychological treatment.

During World War II, it was common knowledge that many servicemen experienced cramp under combat stress and continued with their duties, albeit uncomfortably.

1941: KINNEAR WILSON IN THE UNITED STATES

When Kinnear Wilson reviewed the cramp literature, he emphasised the emotional aspects mentioned by previous authorities. He cited Culpin (1931), who found 31 of his 41 subjects were psychoneurotic. Wilson noted that some cramp subjects had no symptoms of nervousness at all. He distinguished between pre-existing neurotic temperament and the influence of stress as an antecedent. He identified the psychoneurotic symptoms that sometimes manifested after the onset of cramp, in which case they represented distress secondary to disability or pain.

Kinnear Wilson also postulated a writing centre and saw it as mal-functioning, 'deranged from above, at its own level and from below'. 'From above' referred to excitants or depressants of a psychological kind, namely apprehension, fear, anxiety, self-consciousness, mental strain, some feeling of injustice, a grudge or a lack of willpower in a responsible position. Onset was determined by anxiety of one kind or another: business, financial, domestic or other worries, sudden extra strains and states of poor health. 'At its own level' might refer to a 'neuropathic' or 'psychopathic' constitution or a state of irritable weakness, a nervous constitution that broke down under physical or emotional stress, now termed a 'personal vulnerability'. 'From below' implied a mechanism whereby local conditions in the limb handicapped movement by exerting an inhibitory effect. He noted that a number of local factors, including neuralgia, neuritis, rheuma-tism, injury and sprain, were common. Predisposing and exciting determinants did not apply all round and multiple causation had to be admitted.

Kinnear Wilson did not expect cramp to have a morbid anatomy, at least none able to be laid bare by techniques available at that time.

1947: PAI IN GREAT BRITAIN

Narashima Pai, a psychiatrist, based his study on 1880 patients who were hospitalised with neuropsychiatric symptoms between 1941 and 1946. These included returned servicemen who had been recruited from skilled, semi-skilled and unskilled occupations as well as mem-bers of the learned professions: a bank manager, some novelists, jour-nalists, solicitors, a bibliographer, a trainer of wild animals and an 'approved candidate for parliament' (Pai 1947). Only six were clerks and 97 per cent were not clerical workers. Many were too ill to write anything. Their average age was 24.1 years and 171 of them exhibit-ed a disturbance in co-ordination.

Pai divided them into those who were very anxious, those suf-fering from chronic and mild neurosis and those who were suffering from organic diseases of the nervous system. Most patients exhibit-ed anxiety, hysteria or depression. Pai solved his difficulties with classification by introducing his own, 'tremulous, spastic and ataxic', which he attributed to anxiety, neurosis and hysteria, respectively. In this context, ataxic referred to a disorder of control of the required movements.

Pai thought that the importance of the subject lay in the fact that, in the United Kingdom, some cramps had been included among the dangerous trades for the purpose of workers' compensation. In the United States and France, where employers did not pay for disability, the incidence of cramp was negligible. Pai took the position that cramp was 'only a symptom' of neurosis and suggested calling it a 'writing disturbance'. While physicians who postulated a physiological cause for the symptom prescribed complete rest and abstention from writing, Pai noted that French neuropsychiatrists advocated more active therapies, summed up in Janet's admirable words, 'education, excitation and guidance'. Pai reviewed the work of Jelliffe, a neurologist, who found the spastic form of cramp, alone or with tremors, accounted for 40 per cent of his cases. He thought the disorder to be a manifestation of 'a disorientated cortical control', reminiscent of the finding of 'nervous breakdown' by the Departmental Committee of 1911. Pai imitated Radovice, who first recommended atropine, a drug given for Parkinson's disease, making himself an advocate of treating a symptom that suggested a disease as if it was disease itself.

PSYCHOLOGISTS AND PSYCHIATRISTS

Papers by psychologists and psychiatrists advanced a behavioural approach and claimed some successes, which, in the absence of comparison with untreated control subjects, might have been spontaneous remissions (Liversedge & Sylvester 1955). Those who wrote of cures by psychotherapy or psychoanalysis rarely, if ever, identified the issues in the patients' lives that had been targeted for re-evaluation.

It is rarely made clear by those who practise it whether having psychotherapy meant that the patients were simply allowed to talk of what they wanted, or if specific issues were the focus of attention. Like the concept of treatment, which covers any and every doctor–patient contact, the content of psychotherapy, compared with other conversations, has remained obscure.

Sylvester, Liversedge and Beech worked at the Institute of Psychiatry in London at a time when the behavioural psychologist Hans Eysenck was influential there. Conditioning techniques were applied in 39 of their 56 cases. Twenty-nine were thought to be cured but five relapsed. Their patients reported that their anxiety was caused by cramp and that they were concerned for their future earning power. No doubt this was the case but, irrespective of that protestation, 15 were noted to have extraneous sources of anxiety and 20 others (about 30 per cent) 'abnormal traits' and a 'psycho-neurotically fertile' history (Sylvester & Liversedge 1960).

Sylvester and Liversedge acknowledged the numerous successes reported with psychoanalytic treatment, but also its failures. Beech's treatment was based on a behavioural therapy called 'reciprocal inhibition' combined with listening, and he claimed modest success (Beech 1960).

Crisp and Moldofsky (1965), both psychiatrists, viewed cramp as a 'psychosomatic disorder' before somatoform disorders were differentiated from that category. They studied seven patients longitudinally and quantified some aspects of their transference to the therapist during treatment. Transference is the patient's attitude to the doctor. Patients with somatoform disorders initially spend a good deal of their time with doctors defending their right to be seen as physically rather than psychologically ill.

On the basis of self-rating scales, all the patients in their series responded favourably and six reported a favourable response outside of writing.

In Berlin, 58 writers' cramp subjects were hospitalised as in-patients and treated with psychotherapy. On discharge 74.1 per cent of them reported that they felt improved. However, at follow-up some weeks later, only 17 per cent were demonstrably improved and only 38 per cent were feeling better than they had before they went into hospital for this elaborate and expensive remedy (Schultze & Jacob 1988).

1982: SHEEHY AND MARSDEN

In 1982 a neurologist and neuropsychiatrist jointly published a seriously flawed paper in *Brain,* a prestigious journal of neurology (Sheehy & Marsden 1982). It became influential for reasons that were not apparent from its research base and its conclusions do not reflect its content.

The paper was a small study of 29 subjects with writers' cramp, none of whom were vocational writers. They included a hairdresser, a greengrocer, a waitress, a barmaid, a research psychologist, a production line worker, a teacher and an industrial scientist, as well as a dozen clerks, five accountants, four students and four typists.

Eight of the subjects had presented to a university department of neurology with dystonic symptoms and 21 with simple cramp.

During the course of the investigation, eight more subjects 'progressed' to having dystonic symptoms. This meant that 13 continued to describe their difficulties as 'aching', 'clumsiness', 'muscular spasm' and apparent 'inco-ordination' and did not develop dystonic symptoms at all. In spite of these mixed and contradictory findings concerning dystonic symptoms, the authors' conclusion was that cramp was an idiopathic focal dystonia. 'Idiopathic' means that doctors do not know its cause, while 'dystonia' means abnormal muscle tone. Dystonia can be spastic, presenting as spasm or cramp, or flaccid like palsy. In neurology, each phenomenon suggests a different pathological basis.

Sheehy and Marsden believed that they demonstrated the absence of gross psychiatric disorder in their sample by using an established questionnaire, *Present State Examination* (PSE), which they described as a validated interview technique for the presence and severity of psychiatric symptoms. PSE does not identify somatization and will not identify hysteria, in which a person's mental state is characterised by denial of untoward affects and is apparently normal, nor will it identify mild psychological distress. They did note that four of their cases had obvious psychological precipitants, mostly bereavements and health impairments.

On the basis of their investigation, Sheehy and Marsden concluded that cramp was not associated with psychiatric disorder. They further concluded that writers' cramp was not a psychological disturbance but a physical illness, even though no pathology had ever been demonstrated. They went on to postulate an origin in the basal ganglia, arguing that there was a similarity between some of the symptoms of writers' cramp and those of neurological diseases involving lesions in the basal ganglia. On the basis of this analogy, they treated their subjects as if they had Parkinson's disease (Lang et al. 1982). Sheehy and Marsden took the position that Gowers' use of the term 'neurosis' was in accordance with what they believed to be 'the nineteenth century use of the term, a physical disease with no discernible cause'.

This interpretation of Gowers' position on the morbid anatomy of neurosis attracted criticism (*Lancet* 1982). It was also suggested that, if the theory of Sheehy and Marsden implied discrete neurological lesions, it would be difficult to account for cramp sometimes being cured by hypnotherapy (Beeson & Walker 1983). The paper also prompted concern about the dangers of arguing from analogy and the suggestion was made that Sheehy and Marsden had made it even harder for neurologists to refer patients to a psychiatrist (Hudgson 1982).

Sheehy and Marsden challenged the neurological establishment to adopt their formulation and, after some demur, the major school of British neurologists took up their model. British psychiatrists, including authors of the *Oxford Textbook of Psychiatry* (2nd edn), were co-opted in support, as Marsden had been influential in training many of them. Cramp, along with spasmodic torticollis, the Gilles de la Tourette syndrome, tics and Parkinson's disease are all classified as 'movement disorders' within a chapter on organic psychiatry (Gelder et al. 1991).

Lishman (1980) pointed out that psychogenic theories have been varied, relating to psychodynamic or personality configurations, but there seemed to be little indication that the disorder was of a psychiatric nature. He found the firmest evidence in favour of emotional causation to be negative in character as it was indeed hard to conceive of an organic disorder in which movements were impaired when they involved a set of co-ordinated acts performed for one purpose but remained unaffected when making the same movements for another purpose. (It was generally known that some cramp subjects who could not use a typewriter could still play the piano.) He found organic theories to be just as inferential as the psychological and he declined to draw the syndrome into neurological jurisdiction.

Lord Brain edited his own textbook, *Diseases of the Nervous System,* from its first edition to its seventh. He classified cramp as an occupational neurosis, but separately from hysteria. In the ninth edition, Lord Walton, at that time a sole editor, resisted the analysis of Sheehy and Marsden with a critical commentary on the paper (Walton 1985). The tenth edition, now called *Brain's Diseases of the Nervous System,* came under the editorship of multiple authors and omitted the occupational neuroses altogether (Walton et al. 1993). The new editors adopted the position that, as there was no excessive psychiatric morbidity, writers' cramp should fall into the spectrum of idiopathic dystonias.

Placing occupational cramp among other dystonias gave therapeutic jurisdiction to neurologists, and this spawned another set of novel interventions. By general agreement, there was no pathology to be found in the brains of cramp subjects. Yet some accepted analogies with Parkinson's disease and with lesions of the basal ganglia and took the analogy one step further, intervening on behalf of such a condition. This reasoning resulted in the application of remedies that would have been unthinkable had the symptoms been seen as somatization or psychogenic.

Reasoning from analogy encouraged neurosurgeons to intervene with stereotactic surgery to ablate various parts of the brain. (Ablate is a medical euphemism for destroy.) Curiously, the section of the brain needing ablation in writers' cramp varied with the operating surgeon and with the country in which the surgery was being performed. In Poland the operation is described as thalotomy; in France, surgeons perform a 'préfrontal topectomy' (Seigfreid et al. 1969; Mempel et al. 1986; Rouquier 1951).

More recently there has been a vogue for injecting the muscles affected by cramps with dilute botulinus toxin (Tim & Massey 1992; Lees et al. 1992). The symptomatology makes it hard to justify, on theoretical grounds, why a local treatment, an injection into a seemingly affected muscle to which symptoms are being referred, might help the patient. In spite of this, some patients recover. Botulinus toxin is an effective remedy for some dystonias of focal origin. It also enjoys popularity in plastic surgery for ironing out wrinkles.

FROM 1955: HUNTER'S *THE DISEASES OF OCCUPATIONS*

In the United Kingdom, *The Diseases of Occupations* has been the authoritative text on occupational health since its first publication in 1955. It has always had a foot in each camp and its analysis has vacillated like the homage of the Vicar of Bray. Donald Hunter himself recognised cramp to be a neurosis, yet he classified it in a section called 'Diseases due to physical agents', consistent with UK legislation that covered dangerous trades but not consistent with the psychogenic theory of neurosis. This is an example of how legal definitions of medical problems serve to confuse doctors and their treatments. By 1955 about a hundred occupations were considered dangerous. The list grew with each edition until no job was spared.

In its first edition (1955), Hunter described occupational cramps as 'a group of psychoneuroses in which certain symptoms are excited by the attempt to perform a customary act involving an oft-repeated muscular action ... known as craft palsies, occupational palsies and professional spasms'.

The first to third editions listed numerous cramps, categorising them primarily by the occupation of the subject and secondarily by their clinical features, as if the author was under the impression that each was a different form of the disorder (Hunter 1955, 1957, 1962). Hunter was aware that workplace characteristics such as the type of keys, length of service, hours of work and bad style were not the antecedents of cramp. He saw, as antecedents, personal factors, temperamental instability, a nervous temperament, neurasthenia and a highly-strung disposition, attributes 'clearly those of the psychoneurotic person who shows pathological anxiety'.

In Hunter's view, the condition was clearly of central origin and this hypothesis was supported by the fact that symptoms developed in the unused hand of people whose occupational tasks involved the use of only one hand.

In the fourth and fifth editions of his textbook (1969, 1971), Hunter's perspective was reversed. He wrote that most of the occupations in which cramp was reported involved rapid repetitive movements of short range, by one or both hands. But this observation was contradicted on the same pages by his list of 40 occupations in which he had seen cramp develop. Hunter's list included tailors, drapers, hairdressers, ironers, orchestra conductors, waiters and florists. Many had not performed rapid repetitive movements such as those required for writing or for Morse telegraphy. Rather than seeing this material as evidence against causation by task, he ignored the dissonant data. In the later editions, Hunter described only writers' and telegraphists' cramp rather then the array of cramps, which had seemed so different from each other as to need separate classification in earlier times.

In 1987 the book became *Hunter's Diseases of Occupation*, with new editors who came under the influence of a set of theories developed in Australia.

1964–75: OCCUPATIONAL CERVICO-BRACHIAL DISORDER

In 1964 the Japan Association of Occupational Health became concerned with occupational health and decided to investigate the incidence of neck and arm problems in offices and factories. The Association designed a questionnaire to document symptoms in the daily lives of working people. The resulting conglomeration of symptoms was labelled variously as cervico-brachial syndrome, cervical syndrome or thoracic outlet syndrome, and the Association proposed calling this new disease occupational cervico-brachial disorder (OCBD) and attributing it to 'new technology' (Maeda 1977). Across the board, ten per cent of people complained of fatigue at work, with the incidence of complaints being highest in those involved in assembly-line tasks (20.9 per cent) and lowest among management staff (4.0 per cent). An epidemic of neck and arm symptoms followed this occupational health initiative, peaking in 1975. OCBD subjects were noted to be taking tranquillisers and hypnotics and complaining of sleep disturbance, as well as having neck and arm symptoms. Fatigue in the neck, back, arms and eyes, pain, dullness at the back, coldness, numbness and motor disturbances of hand, finger tremor and irregular menstruation were common and were thought to be evidence of a severe stage of this new disorder (Keikenwan 1973).

Japanese medical lore took a very organic view of the syndrome. None of Japan's medical literature touched on vulnerability factors in individuals and it referred only in passing to psychosocial factors in various workplaces. No comment was made on problems in the subjects' lives. The epidemic spread of the disorder following attention being paid to it and the increase in claims lent credence to the notion that the Japanese problem could have been an epidemic of symptoms spread by the ideas implied in its questionnaire.

4

RSI AND INDUSTRIAL RELATIONS

The bureaucracy is a circle from which no one can escape.
Its hierarchy is a hierarchy of knowledge. The top entrusts
the understanding of detail to the lower levels, while the
lower levels credit the top with understanding of the general
and both are mutually deceived.

Karl Marx, *Contribution to the Critique of Hegel's Philosophy of Right*

In the 1980s, occupational cramp reappeared in Australia as repetitive strain injury, or RSI. Its incidence rose rapidly to epidemic proportions and then declined, leaving an endemic disorder and unresolved issues at every level.

Concern for the effects of work conditions involving repetitive movements can be traced back to Freidrich Engels (1820–95), who believed that musculoskeletal disorders resulted from the appalling conditions that he described in the mines and factories of England at the turn of the century.

All of these affectations are clearly explained by the nature of factory work. The operative … must stand the whole time … and this constant mechanical pressure of the upper portions of the body upon spinal column, hips and legs, inevitably produces the results mentioned. (Engels 1845)

Engels' account of the conditions of the working classes of England was as passionate as it was horrifying. Engels devoted his early life and energy to refuting the beliefs of his father, who was a proponent of puritanical pietism, which, in effect, blamed the poor and sick for their own suffering. Engels concluded that pietism worsened such problems by giving doctrinal interpretations based on individual responsibility and in that it supported a reluctance to intervene effectively in social deprivation. The same notion of external cause underpinned the injury model of workplace symptoms and determined the angry criticism towards the application of the somatization model. It was seen as blaming the victim. Howard Waitzkin (1981), a medically qualified sociologist, drew attention to Engels' beliefs and endorsed their content.

> The insight that chronic musculoskeletal disorders could result from unchanging posture or small, repetitive movements seems simple enough. Yet this source of illness, which is quite different from a specific accident or exposure to a toxic substance, has entered occupational medicine as a serious concern only in the last two decades.

OCCUPATIONAL HEALTH AND SAFETY

Concern about occupational health and safety (OHS) had been developing in the industrialised world since the early 1960s. Both had been neglected during the Depression, World War II and its aftermath. This interest could be seen as part of a social movement that accommodated concern for environmental issues and public health. It culminated in formation of institutions and OHS legislation in many Western countries. Much concern has been expressed about both the effectiveness and rationality of the legislation that was being passed in the United States (Coye et al. 1984; Jasanoff 1989). A major focus was said to be the introduction of worker-appointed safety representatives (Creighton 1982).

A similar upsurge in interest in OHS had occurred in the United Kingdom, while the impact of recession and unemployment was said to have dampened enthusiasm. Legitimate concerns developed about the management of human capital as increasing and ever-changing demands were being made on workers to be retrained and educated. By the early 1990s, a flurry of directives concerning standards for manual workers had started to emerge from the European Community offices in Brussels. These were based on Australian ideas.

The occupational health movement again came to include the

instrumental use of occupational health to drive an industrial relations agenda. A medical dissertation of what was safe needed to be
devised and used to accommodate its needs. Industrial relations matters had to be turned into health issues.

The medical profession was invited into the workplace and doctors were encouraged to medicalise the consequences of fatigue, discomfort and poor management as if they were physical injuries to
arms. Workers who experienced problems had less need of union delegates to sort them out.

The unions failed to recognise that they were handing over, as if
on a platter, their traditional responsibilities and making their own
role redundant. The medical certificate became the currency of negotiation but it turned out to be an ineffective way of communicating
dissatisfaction with a state of affairs. Medicalisation of industrial relations contributed to a fall in union membership a few years later.

When the occupational stress epidemic replaced the RSI epidemic in the early 1990s, the profession was already poised to medicalise
as psychological injury the consequences of very hurtful abrasive and
dysfunctional relationships as well as the stresses of overwork and
understaffing. The distressed worker who rang his or her union was
advised to go to the doctor to get a certificate. The interpersonal
behaviours that had caused stress remained unchecked. The rehabilitation provider arrived on the scene some weeks later and replaced
the shop steward as the one who articulated and negotiated the concerns of the worker.

Certain strategic events and activities marked the construction of
this new knowledge and its legitimation in New South Wales,
Victoria and the Australian Commonwealth sector of employment.

THE DEVELOPMENT OF THE
CONSTRUCTION OF RSI

Unions had little room to manoeuvre for improvements in wages and
hours during the period of wage indexation, 1978–81, so they
focused on the long-neglected issue of health and safety. Moral
entrepreneurs of health teamed up with unions and enrolled the
major institutions, government, medicine, law and the media.

Trade unions used trusted legal firms to win compensation for
their members. Their lawyers were skilled in identifying medical
experts whose views were likely to be useful, experts who, like
Engels, believed that repetitive activities had a deleterious effect on

the body and that this was the responsibility of the employer. These experts turned their attention to typists and data processing officers (DPOs) and attributed the symptoms of the emerging epidemic to the hypothetical trauma of pressing buttons on an electronic keyboard at the rate of as few as 400 keystrokes an hour. A lesion diagnosis could not be made or postulated in those cases so doctors who became interested in RSI went on to diagnose a great number of lesions to account for a plethora of symptoms.

A relatively small number of physicians and ergonomists were placed in positions where they were able to influence strategic institutions in ways that ultimately brought about an epidemic of work disability.

The union movement, employers, government, judges and experts all played their parts in constructing RSI as an injury. Each assumed that the knowledge of the others who claimed expertise in RSI was based on a secure, scientific foundation, and all were mutually deceived.

THE CONFLATION OF INDUSTRIAL TRAUMA AND OCCUPATION NEUROSIS

The knowledge that injuries can be caused by occupational tasks was not new. Ramazzini (1700), Donald Hunter and Nortin Hadler (1984, 1986) documented the symptoms, signs and natural histories of the trauma-induced conditions. Hadler noted that, with rare exceptions, these lesions were preceded by events that involved external force. Diagnosis was seldom at issue and the management was well described in the surgical literature. Prophylaxis was possible and recourse to workers' compensation programs was efficient. Such injuries, however, occurred in tissues that had been traumatised by use, they related to the quantum of trauma suffered, they were localised, they recovered with rest and they ran a familiar course.

RSI was not an epidemic of this kind of injury. The Australian RSI was more diffuse and accounted for much more dense work disability, and it persisted for longer periods. It did not respond to rest or the remedies that were known to be effective for disorders of traumatic origin.

The notion of repetitive strain injuries and their North American counterparts, cumulative trauma disorders (CTDs), had its roots in two distinct lines of literature: traumatic rheumatology and the occupation neuroses. The cause of CTDs, by its inherently circular definition, is cumulative trauma. But those who published about RSI and CTDs cited the literature concerning traumatic lesions haphazardly with the literature of functional disorders. They seemed unaware that mental events caused the occupation neuroses and that physical forces caused traumatic lesions.

RSI and CTDs were of strategic interest, not only to the OHS lobby, but also to workers, policy makers and activists who wanted safer, healthier workplaces and more supportive industrial arrangements. The very words 'injury' and 'disorder' implied that they were legitimately the province of medicine and that there was a medical, that is, clinical-science-based, justification for limiting any worker's output.

As with RSI in Australia, the prevention of CTDs attracted research funds and a scientific community in the United States. Monitoring these disorders and investigating outbreaks of them were part of the program for the National Institute of Occupational Safety and Health (NIOSH), which was one of the Centers for Disease Control. These centres played their share in legitimating cumulative trauma disorder by prosecuting those employers who fell victim to it.

Poorly defined syndromes with slow recovery rates were attributed to the effects of cumulative trauma. The clinical picture comprised a variety of symptoms, pain and tingling, and abnormal sensations such as temperature changes or feeling swollen or clumsy. These were combined with motor weakness, occasionally palsy, but more often an inability to perform the specific task that was being held responsible for their development. Symptoms were different in every case and, because of this, RSI attracted a large number of diagnostic labels and pathological speculations. Nor was the mode of onset a constant. These problems were unresponsive to physical therapies and were accompanied by emotional distress or by complacent indifference. Distress was reported to be the consequence of the injury but, on inquiry, stressful events had preceded the development of symptoms.

This diagnostic confusion had two important consequences. First, clinicians failed to diagnose functional syndromes, making type I errors, missing a positive diagnosis. Second, they diagnosed the disease states that these syndromes resembled and thus made type II errors. They diagnosed conditions which these patients did not suffer from. The problem was compounded when, having made a type II error and having put the patient unnecessarily in the sick role, treating physicians intervened clinically on behalf of hypothetical disease entities (Hadler 1992). Treatments proliferated because of this confusion. Those given within an injury framework were unsuccessful.

The conflation of the two models of explanation inspired researchers to inquire into personal attributes of subjects who had been diagnosed as having entrapment neuropathies (Armstrong & Chaffin 1979). These authors did not explain exactly how personal attributes could change connective tissues. Surgeons attributed various entrapment neuropathies to the 'cumulative trauma-induced' but still hypothetical thickening of tendon sheaths said to be causing the compromise of peripheral nerves. Unsuccessful surgical interventions were legitimated by court decisions, in the face of well-acknowledged and available information that carpal tunnel syndrome, even loosely defined as it is in virtually all the American literature, was not related to workplace factors and was not a cumulative trauma disorder (Hadler 1993). No sanctions could be considered against those who performed unsuccessful surgery, as a respectable body of medical opinion could always be found to support such interventions. The use of non-specific criteria to diagnose median nerve entrapment had already been legitimated, as early as 1963, in a standard textbook by a contemporary of Lord Brain's, Sir Francis Walshe (1963). Median nerve entrapment is rare, although transient nocturnal symptoms involving the territory of the median nerve are extremely common. The condition with discrete symptoms always responds to surgery (Brain 1947; Stevens et al. 1988). Some American states have created legal definitions of carpal tunnel syndrome that are not congruent with medical criteria for their diagnosis. These conditions do not submit to surgical remedies.

1961–79: TENOSYNOVITIS

Velpeau first used the term 'tenosynovitis' in 1818. In Australia in 1961, Perrot drew attention to what he termed 'the large variety of occupational trauma that occurred in industrial workers'. He believed that the primary cause of tenosynovitis was the excessive use of the same sets of muscles and that prevention could and should be achieved by task alteration and rest breaks. He had some measurable influence, as Workers' Compensation Commission statistics reveal a rise in the incidence of reporting of tenosynovitis in New South Wales in 1963–64. Then it fell back again.

A decade later, Ferguson (1971b) published on what he called 'repetition injuries' in process workers and, in the same year, he reported on telegraphists' cramp, noting the large discrepancy in its incidence between Victoria and New South Wales (Ferguson 1971a). This drew editorial comment in the *British Medical Journal* (1972) to the effect that cramp seemed to be very common in Australia.

In 1972 Welsh described both the physiological and psychological conditions predisposing to what he called tenosynovitis.

In 1976 an industrial health group established at the Liverpool Women's Health Centre in New South Wales published a booklet, *Your Job, His Profits or Your Life,* in which information on tenosynovitis was documented. The Workers' Health Action Group was started in Victoria (NOHSC 1986c) and the term 'teno' came into use. The progression of the notion of tenosynovitis to RSI can be traced back to the activities of the Workers' Health Centre at Lidcombe, NSW.

1979: TENOSYNOVITIS, WALKER AND THE WORKERS' HEALTH CENTRE

In 1979, Dr Jim Walker of the Workers' Health Centre reported in *New Doctor* on 'tenosynovitis and/or carpal tunnel syndrome' in 'Tenosynovitis: A Crippling New Epidemic in Industry'. *New Doctor* is published by the Doctors' Reform Society and is not a refereed medical journal.

This publication promoted the notion that one could have a long, disabling and compensable condition if one were experiencing a variety of symptoms in the arms. Walker postulated that

the cause of inflammation may be exhaustion of the supply of synovial fluid (which lubricates the tendons) because the sheer number of movements of the tendons overwhelms secretory capacity ... that the frictional heat generated by so much activity breaks down the synovial fluid producing a toxic inflammatory by-product.

Walker did not cite any previous reports of sporadic or epidemic cases of a non-recovering tenosynovitis with such extensive manifestations and distribution. Nor did he cite any evidence that drying up could or did occur. His assertions contradicted the accepted view that irritation increased the circulation of blood supply and that this caused overproduction of synovial fluid with the net result being an effusion, not a drying up. Walker's formulation of a hypothetical traumatic condition made the reporting of symptoms compensable under legislation that existed at the time.

In so naming this prolonged symptomatology, Walker described a new disease. He had to extend the meaning of tenosynovitis to cover a condition that did not behave like an 'itis', or inflammation. Tenosynovitis, as reported in textbooks, was a localised problem of brief duration, one that recovered with rest and with specific treatments appropriate to an inflammation. Sometimes the inflammation scarred the tendon sheath and caused contraction.

The Workers' Health Centre catered for manual and clerical workers rather than a cross-section of the community. Walker believed most workers continued working 'because of financial reasons and fear of getting sacked if they went off sick' and that the 'usual pattern was that they go off work on compensation and many are never able to work again'. Of those who had been off work, half reported that their symptoms returned on their first day back and most of them had to go off again.

Walker contested the diagnoses made by his patients' family doctors. Their opinions did not always accord with his. He distrusted management, which, he believed, told workers the disease was 'in them'. He suggested that this was an attempt to 'con' the worker into believing the symptoms were not caused by the work process.

Walker's paper noted the use of psychotropic (mind-directed or mind-altering) medication among his patients. When he asked his patients which treatments had helped the most, 'none at all' and 'rest' were the most common answers. Walker reported that a wide variety of treatments were used for this condition and noted its resistance not only to surgery but also to rest, support, slings, plaster, ultrasound, cortisone injection, physiotherapy involving exercises, faradic, hot wax baths and ultrasound, operations and tablets, including indomethacin, butazolidine, paracetamol and dextropropoxyphene hydrochloride.

Nineteen out of 45 of Walker's surveyed patients had been operated on at least once for what they were told was carpal tunnel syndrome. Sixteen had been told that the operation would cure them, but only one had been cured. Thirteen of the 19 said that they felt the operation had made them worse and 11 said they felt that it had permanently crippled them. Only three of those who had been given the operation were back working.

Walker's hypothesis for failure of the release operation was complex. He believed that there was 'simple carpal tunnel syndrome' and 'carpal tunnel syndrome secondary to tenosynovitis'. He believed that 'surgery was rarely curative in tenosynovitis' because it promoted adhesions and excessive scar tissue that only further compromised tendon function.

The influence of Walker's theories was remarkable. They became the subject of the *Workers' Health Centre Information Leaflet No. 1* (1982) and the acknowledged source of information for OHS policies and manuals. The Workers' Health Centre sent speakers to RSI awareness seminars, made liaison with the Amalgamated Metal Workers' and Shipwrights Union (AMWSU) and influenced the policy of the manufacturing unions. The Workers' Health Centre, to its credit, listed a number of conditions in arms that were not RSI. These included thoracic outlet syndrome, various systemic diseases and arthritis. Eighty-six out of their 89 cases were 'chronic' and the Workers' Health Centre reported that the specialists to whom they referred their patients found that most people with such injuries were slow to recover.

The Workers' Health Centre became an activist organisation in the interests of OHS and it made a well-publicised submission to the Williams Commission, a public inquiry into occupational health established in New South Wales in 1979.

The Williams Commission adopted the principles of the Robens Committee in England to the effect that there was a commonality of interest in health and safety (Robens 1970–72; Williams 1981). Williams reported in 1981 and the NSW *Occupational Health and Safety Act 1983* was loosely based on those recommendations (Robinson 1986).

The Centre also distributed a quarterly newsletter and a detailed pamphlet, *Tenosynovitis and Other Occupational Over-Use Injuries: Information for Doctors and Health Workers* (1982). This document advised doctors on how to take a history of precipitating factors and gave advice on the periods when tenosynovitis was more likely to occur. This was noted to be on return from holidays and with increases in work rate. The causes of 'teno' were said to be seating, lack of appropriate furniture, machinery, tools, posture, physical movements, static muscle loading and the neck being in flexion or hyperextension.

Doctors participating in the diagnosis of these conditions were advised to become involved in prevention strategies, to remove workers complaining of symptoms from the workplace and to treat them and provide certificates for compensation. Doctors were advised not to send workers back while they were still being treated. Workers were turned into patients, then into claimants for a condition for which there was apparently no medical remedy. Access to domestic, legal and financial help was advertised. The Workers' Health Centre saw many more cases in 1979 (Taylor et al. 1982).

Pamphlets, so called 'grey literature', played a prominent role in the coming epidemic of disability. Patients read the 'guides to prevention' in doctors' waiting rooms. Educated in this way, they recited their symptoms, reporting the causal attributions they had learnt and, in this way, educated the doctors from whom they sought medicolegal reports. As Shorter (1992) has described in his history of psychosomatic symptoms over 200 years, the doctor's paradigm, or model of explanation, followed patients' ideas of what was wrong with them. Medical knowledge continued to be constructed out of the anxieties of laymen and workers and not out of scientific information.

Walker's hypothesis had no support in conventional medicine, but it came to pass for common knowledge. His formulations entered the medicolegal reports of physicians, surgeons and occupational health specialists, many of whom adopted the concept of a non-recovering teno as if it was well-established medical knowledge.

The construction tenosynovitis reappeared as 'muscular repetition injury' in *Repetition Injury in Process Workers,* the proceedings of a conference in Victoria, which was attended by Workers' Health Centre employees. It dictated exactly how workers could be encouraged to make claims for symptoms that they had formerly regarded as trivial (AMWSU 1983):

Two women ... initially said that they didn't have tenosynovitis, but as we started talking about their job it came out that they had all the symptoms; swollen hands at night, pain, tingling in the hands and one of them had pain in her neck. They also talked about how heavy their particular process was and how their work was the heaviest, so no one would want their jobs and they would be the only ones who would want to rotate.

Barbara McPhee, a physiotherapist, had taken up the issue of preventing tenosynovitis in the late 1970s. She worked with Professor David Ferguson in the Commonwealth Institute of Occupational

Health and she had been presenting papers on posture and keyboard work for years (McPhee 1979, 1980a, 1980b). McPhee came into possession of reports by the ergonomists who had been involved in both the Finnish and Japanese epidemics of arm symptoms, all of which concerned workplace pain and its assumed causes. These ergonomists' interpretations of 'tenosynovitis and related neck conditions' were to contribute to the voluminous literature of RSI.

In 1980, practitioners of the newly emergent disciplines of ergonomics and safety science were claiming expertise in the prevention of repetition strains. Ergonomists had come from disparate disciplines, including public health, mechanical engineering, psychology, occupational therapy and occupational medicine (Howie & Wyatt 1985). Few had formal training or qualifications in ergonomics, a discipline that in the UK covers all aspects of work, not just the mechanical ones. In Australia, ergonomics seemed to be limited to the physical aspects of the industrial production process.

In an introduction to a batch of contemporary ergonomists' publications in 1987, at the height of the epidemic, Jim Brassil, chair of WorkSafe, cited what he called 'valuable advice from the Ergonomics Society of Australia and New Zealand'. He informed the reader about how ergonomics had been applied over the previous 15 years to investigate and reduce RSI (Stevenson 1987).

Stevenson, an ergonomist, was Associate Professor and Director of the Centre for Safety Science at the University of New South Wales and had served on the RSI Committee of the NSW Department of Industrial Relations (where Nolan and Elenor were employed), on the Standards Association of Australia (where he had produced the report which he frequently cited) and on the National Occupational Health and Safety Commission, WorkSafe Australia. He was also convenor of the RSI Special Interest Group of the Ergonomics Society of Australia.

1981: THE RANK ELECTRIC DISPUTE

In 1979 the AMWSU was the first union to appoint a full-time safety officer. The AMWSU represented the workers at the Rank-General Electric plant at Notting Hill in Victoria, where a strike occurred in the winter of 1981. The company wanted to dismiss seven women who claimed to be disabled by tenosynovitis and what was being called, at that place, repetition injury (Creighton & Micallef 1983).

This was the first overt conflict about arm symptoms. In 1980 Rank Electric had investigated work practices with a view to introducing modifications to minimise repetitive movements. There had been a rapid rise in the incidence of tenosynovitis at this plant from 8 cases in 1977 to 39 in 1980 to 54 in 1981. In 1983, two years after the supposedly preventative measures had been introduced after the industrial dispute, 90 per cent of injuries at the plant were for conditions that were being called overuse problems.

The AMWSU took the position that GPs had little idea how to treat overuse conditions, so affected workers were referred 'for rehabilitation' to an industrial rehabilitation clinic. The strike was settled on the basis that there was to be an ongoing ergonomic survey to study the extent of RSI and how to reorganise the industrial process with a view to preventing it. The AMWSU agreed to allow their members to return to work in return for a promise to institute injury awareness, job redesign and rotation and to refrain from discouraging women from getting rehabilitated by a particular specialist who was designated as 'the company nominated doctor'. Compensable sick roles were defined for the symptomatic workers on the basis that tenosynovitis was a work-caused injury. At the same time, negotiations were being undertaken to change work practices.

The plant was hard hit by the recession and there were redundancies and dismissals in 1982 and 1983. These included the remaining affected workers, those who had not already left work for other reasons.

1981: THE OCCUPATIONAL HEALTH AND SAFETY UNIT

In June 1981 the Australian Council of Trade Unions (ACTU) and the Victorian Trades Hall Council (VTHC) set up an Occupational Health and Safety Unit (OHSU) 'to provide an information service to unions, to review existing occupational health hazards, to initiate surveys and to make liaison with various authorities and to conduct research'.

In early 1981, before anyone had ever heard of RSI, repetitive or repetition strain injuries, the ACTU/VTHC started to publish the *Health and Safety Bulletin* which, in its very first edition, advised that it was developing a plan for action to reduce tenosynovitis and other overuse injuries (Mathews & Calabrese 1981a).

1981: INVOLVEMENT OF
THE CLERICAL UNIONS

Although repetitive strain injuries were first seen in metal workers, it was the activity of white-collar unions that transformed RSI into a major industrial issue. In 1981 the Federated Clerks' Union (FCU) took up the issue of keyboard and visual display unit (VDU) safety. The leaders of the clerical unions took the position that the introduction of highly productive word-processing technology meant that some of their members would become redundant.

In the late 1970s, British workers had been concerned about the safety aspects of VDU screens, but they had not worried about keyboards. RSI first appeared in England eight years after the introduction of word processors. In the United States, CTDs became an issue in 1986, eight or more years after the introduction of word processors, and an outbreak of arm symptoms followed the introduction of strategies to prevent work-related diseases and injuries.

Curtailing productivity increases seemed to be an effective way of securing jobs, so limits to output needed to be set. There was a risk that computer sweatshops would develop with data input personnel operating in mindless boredom as extensions of machines, performing tasks that were meaningless to them. This concern was highlighted by a British ergonomist, Brian Pearce, who had considerable experience of workplace evaluation. Pearce described the office of the Internal Revenue Service in Brook Haven on Long Island, New York, as it appeared in 1986. DPOs were served by trolley and did their work wearing headphones, listening to radio soaps. RSI was unknown in that workplace until preventative strategies reached it two or three years later. Improvements to work conditions could have been justified in the interests of humanity and efficiency without promoting symptoms and medicalising them (Pearce 1992).

The Federated Clerks' Union covered the Australian Taxation Office (ATO), an office that was strategically positioned to exert pressure on the government. It determined the coercive way that health came to be used in mediating industrial relations.

Grievances among DPOs went back to 1979, when they started filing workers' compensation claims for tenosynovitis. They wanted to safeguard data input jobs that were coming under pressure from increasing electronic submission of taxation returns. They claimed that workloads were increasing and that they did not want to work overtime. They also did not want seasonal or part-time staff to be employed. They wanted to limit their output to 10 000 keystrokes an hour as these were performed with one hand.

The union's position was that tenosynovitis in Data Processing Officers was caused by work rates and ergonomic factors. Two doctors were invited to investigate symptoms, which were presumptively termed occupational injuries and illnesses.

1981: CUMPSTON AND TAYLOR

In Victoria, the notion that keyboard work caused RSI first appeared in 1981 in a smudged, blotchy, nine-page, typewritten document, one copy of which has survived in the archives of the Commonwealth Department of Health. This report by two doctors was to spawn hundreds of thousands of court actions worldwide. Dr Alan G. Cumpston, then the Acting Medical Services Adviser on Occupational Health, Commonwealth Department of Health, represented the government and Dr Richard Taylor, Research Associate in the Department of Social and Preventative Medicine at Monash University, represented the union.

The technique of making inquiries by questionnaire may have some virtue but it is not without risk. In 1911 the Postal Telegraph Clerks' Association had administered a questionnaire during an inquiry and 60 per cent of the workforce reported symptoms. The Japan Association of Occupational Health had administered a questionnaire in 1972 and had named symptoms 'occupational cervico-brachial disorder' (OCBD). This precipitated an epidemic of symptoms and claims under that rubric (Keikenwan 1973; Maeda 1977) As in the United Kingdom and Japan, Cumpston and Taylor's questionnaire converted the discomforts of DPOs into a new traumatic disease.

The Data Processing Officers who responded to the questionnaire had been asked a loaded question: 'Do you have a repetition injury now?' More than 70 per cent of keyboard staff reported that they had some symptoms on a monthly basis, half of the workforce complained of weekly symptoms and about 35 per cent said that symptoms occurred daily. Such symptoms were taken to be either precursors or evidence of 'overuse' diseases such as 'tenosynovitis, tension neck, cervical syndrome, epicondylitis and supraspinatus or bicipital tendinitis'.

Together, Cumpston and Taylor examined 108 of the 133 DPOs in the Taxation Office. They reported 'a high prevalence of repetition injury' among the staff (Cumpston 1981). Cumpston found and reported that 18 of the DPOs were suffering from what he called 'repetition injury' and a further 22 showed 'evidence of muscular strain' in the neck, shoulder, elbow, wrist or hand. He reported that 40 people, or 37 per cent of the workforce, had 'observable occupational injuries' and noted that a further 46 women reported 'effects in their arms or necks as a result of data processing work'. Cumpston found only 22 DPOs who had no work-related symptoms (Taylor 1981). The Australian Public Service Association (APSA) claimed that a quarter of the workforce in the ATO in Melbourne was affected.

None of these conditions had ever been associated with keyboard work before. The notion that typists are liable to develop multiple lesions from their occupational task appeared in the medical literature only after the Australian epidemic, because of extensive misdiagnosis of the numerous conditions with which cramp had historically been confused.

Cumpston reported that 14 DPOs were on workers' compensation and that half of them had been diagnosed by a doctor as having 'tenosynovitis' or 'some similar tendon problem' (Cumpston 1981). Those not at work at the time of the survey were not examined but they were assumed to be the more serious cases of repetition injury.

Cumpston also reported: 'The main cause of repetition injury in the forearm, wrist and hand is too short a cycle time during repetitive movement of the fingers. Other factors are unnecessarily forceful action and prolonged periods of work.' Cumpston found bilateral symptoms in people who performed keyboard work with only one hand. He came to the conclusion that 'The constant handling of documents with the left hand appears to be the reason why signs of muscular strain were frequently found in the left side of the neck and the left shoulder'. In this way Cumpston conferred medical authority to the notion that the physical activities associated with pressing buttons on an electronic keyboard could cause a repetition injury and that turning over papers with the left hand could cause a muscular strain.

Cumpston recommended a keystroke rate of not more than 12 000 per hour on any task. This is the equivalent of a typing speed of 30–40 words per minute with two hands or 60–80 with one hand. There were clear rules in the public sector about status, capability and pay. To be a typist, a person had to be able to type at 60 words a minute, while 80 words or more were expected at senior grades. Stenographers were proficient at higher rates and clerks, who typed only occasionally, needed to be capable of 30 words a minute.

Cumpston's recommendation suggested that long-standing norms were unsafe.

The investigation by Taylor and Cumpston foreshadowed a level of co-operation between the state and doctors able to express expert opinions which suited the demands of unions and stabilised industrial conflict. Opportunities for shop-floor negotiation and resolution were handed unconditionally to medical personnel who were willing to redefine them as medical problems.

Doctors who were prepared to venture opinions on what was medically desirable rather than industrially achievable willingly replaced union organisers. Medical authority resolved an industrial issue. This had one unintended consequence in that it bypassed union activity in white-collar workplaces.

The *Health and Safety Bulletin* related that 'Dr Cumpston's report was so damning that it was adopted by the unions as well'.

The review team of Cumpston and Taylor made 27 specific recommendations, which did not entirely satisfy the union's demands. The dispute was referred for arbitration under the *Public Service Arbitration Act 1920* and 60 days of hearings produced the *Booth Determination* (Booth 1983).

Cumpston gave evidence to this tribunal largely on the issue of how many keystrokes an hour it was safe to perform. Both parties had reservations about the figures and a compromise rate of 11 000 was eventually deemed acceptable.

John Mathews of the ACTU/VTHC gave evidence for the unions. He was the originator of the acronym RSI and the publisher of the *Health and Safety Bulletin*. Mathews was not a medical graduate. A number of Victorian GPs also gave evidence. Their claim to expertise was that they were involved in workers' health activities, treating claimants with RSI as if they had injuries. The Public Service Board called Dr Christopher Browne and Professor David Ferguson. The physiotherapist Barbara McPhee gave evidence on prevention. The Tribunal called Dr Alan Cumpston and Dr William Stone as experts.

Acting Arbitrator Booth encouraged the parties to decide jointly on what they wanted. He then ratified their agreement on training, with management agreeing to take advice from Dr Browne on diagnostic matters and from Ms McPhee on prevention, work allocation procedures, redeployment policy, ergonomics, job rotation, keying time, proficiency allowance, maximum and minimum rates, rest breaks, statistics and shiftwork.

Faced with increasing absenteeism, employers moved to meet union demands regarding workplace conditions. New attribution theories for RSI had to be found, for many affected workers had performed neither the rapid nor the repetitive movements that keyboard work entailed. Doctors were prepared to ascribe causal status to any undesirable aspect of any workplace. RSI was consequently attributed to tissue damage caused by faulty work stations, furniture, equipment, incorrect posture, noise, inactivity, overwork, repetitive work, having worked for too many years, soft touch keyboards, old banger typewriters, the mouse, badly positioned VDUs and to emanations from Black Mountain Tower, the microwave facility overlooking Canberra.

The medical community failed to question the findings that these medical examiners had produced in this unique social context. This failure introduced a falsehood, a canard, into medical and scientific literature. Its introduction and acceptance were to have serious long-term repercussions. A pandemic of arm symptoms followed.

In Australian law, the status of any doctor as an expert could not be challenged. The legal issue would be decided on the plausibility of his opinion. His knowledge of a medical subject was rarely examined in court. There was no legal distinction between the opinions of those who had expert status and of those who claimed expertise in a body of knowledge that had been generated by scientific method.

The issue of RSI and occupational health was taken up in a paramedical journal, *Community Health Studies*, which had published Dr Taylor's report, *Repetition Injury in Process Workers* (Taylor 1981; Taylor & Pitcher 1984). Taylor published in conjunction with Chris Gow and Stephen Corbett, who were described as researchers from the Workers' Health Centre at Lidcombe. The editor of *Community Health Studies*, Neville Hicks, introduced a paper by this group (Taylor et al. 1982) and admitted that it was not that journal's usual policy to publish papers that were 'essentially clinical', but that he wanted

... to provide data to those working in Occupational Health on the diversity of symptoms which may occur as a result of repetitive work, information which is not yet being promoted by other journals in Australia, in the expectation of stimulating more formal epidemiological and sociological studies.

This paper described several cases of 'repetition injury', attributing symptoms to the tasks on which the subjects had been employed.

1982: THE NATIONAL HEALTH AND MEDICAL RESEARCH COUNCIL (NHMRC)

The first nationwide use of the term 'repetition strain injury' and its acronym, RSI, appeared in a document typed in lower case, called *repetition strain injuries: approved guide to occupational health*, which the National Health and Medical Research Council adopted at its meeting in June of 1982, a few months after the decision in *Lashford v Plessey*. It has been extensively cited as the NHMRC *approved guide* and it described 'conditions associated with repetition strain and conditions that might be aggravated by repetitive manual work'. At best, this may have been a consensus document representing various interests, but it was couched in medical terminology. It was much the same in content as the Workers' Health Centre material submitted to the Williams Commission and to the ACTU's *Guidelines for the Prevention of Repetitive Strain Injury,* which were published a couple of months later. The sources of the information in it were not revealed. On the face of it, the *approved guide* was produced by anonymous people in the Commonwealth Department of Health and possibly in the Department of Industrial Relations in New South Wales. The *approved guide* did not provide references for what it recommended. According to John Mathews, the acronym RSI, which the *approved guide* had used, was the brainchild of the ACTU/VTHC health policy unit and was first used in 1981.

The *approved guide to the prevention of repetition strain injuries* was apparently the first 'medical' publication of the injury paradigm of RSI. The prestige of the panel of doctors who comprised the NHMRC was appended to a set of ideas entirely unsupported by evidence.

The *approved guide* endorsed a great deal of information: that assembly, packaging, data processing, typing, machine accounting, stamping, checking, sorting with the constant repetition of movement all imposed a cumulative workload and could cause pain, weakness and impaired functions of the muscles and other soft tissues. This was repetition strain injury and, according to the guide, it was caused by a combination of voluntary and involuntary muscular activity to set the basic posture for the task, with the nature of the posture determining the amount of static muscle load.

Furthermore, RSI was deemed to be caused by the rapid repetition of movements, by the muscular strength required to perform those movements, by inefficient methods of work, by unsuitable hand movements, by the unnecessary use of muscles, by unnecessarily forceful action, and by postures of the arm, trunk or hand which required joints to deviate repeatedly or for long periods from the position of normal function. Also deemed to be causes were unaccustomed work affecting both beginners and workers who came back to work after a break, changes in work patterns, prolonged repetitive work, static loading of muscles and a cycle time that was too short.

The extent to which this was incoherent is demonstrated by the proposed notion that 'muscles might be at their most efficient when the joints are bent'.

The central terms were not defined. There was no definition of what was overuse nor was there sanction of normal use. On a literal interpretation, there was no condition that was not RSI and there was no pain that did not have a work-related, therefore culpable, precursor activity.

This was the legitimated medical start to a campaign whose stated goal was the prevention of a disorder that had not been heard of until this time.

The document itself contained no indication of how it came to be before the Council of the NHMRC and no hint of who might have been its author. Dr Alan Cumpston and Professor David Ferguson were serving on the Occupational Health Committee of the NHMRC at that time. Ferguson came to believe that the *approved guide* was a product of various medical and non-medical persons employed within the Commonwealth Department of Health. There is no experimental evidence for any of the propositions put forward, nor was any ever found after the publication of this material. This document revealed an absence on the part of the NHMRC of any notion of what constituted scientific medicine. It stood testament to the enrolment of the NHMRC in the service of a political goal alien to its role in generating and promoting medical knowledge through research.

In legitimating the notion of repetition strain injury as a condition caused by occupational tasks, the NHMRC became a vector of pandemic. Preventative measures led to disabling symptoms in a workforce whose collective arms were unimpaired until that time.

In publishing and endorsing this document, the NHMRC unleashed an uncontrolled experiment on the community. A group of previously healthy people was told that they were at risk of contracting a preventable disease that could disable them, when there was no such disease. Ethical evaluation of this experiment might have led to the realisation that some of the experimental subjects might suffer greatly and others might never be able to give up the idea that they had been hurt or harmed. Had consideration been given to the predictable consequences of such an experiment, to the literature on the risks of prevention, this experiment, if submitted on a smaller scale, would not have passed the NHMRC's own ethics committees. Experimentation on humans is subject to informed consent. This natural experiment did have one useful result in that it demonstrated the extent to which beliefs about one's body are the causes of somatization.

The injury paradigm of RSI was now sufficiently established, as Latour (1979) might suggest, to acquire a scientific community to undertake research and to recruit practitioners to follow its dictates in their interventions. A review of extensive research funding into RSI by the NHMRC failed to reveal a single grant for a project that was not in the dominant paradigm, nor any that were not based on an assumption that RSI was an injury caused by work.

1982: ACTU DRAFTS POLICY: *GUIDELINES FOR THE PREVENTION OF REPETITIVE STRAIN INJURY*

In the December 1981 issue of its *Health and Safety Bulletin*, the ACTU announced its intention to promote the 'prevention of overuse injuries' in order to get the workplace changes it desired. In August 1982 the promised document, *RSI: Guidelines for the Prevention of Repetitive Strain Injury*, was published (Mathews & Calabrese 1982). It will be referred to as the ACTU's *Guidelines*.

The name, as well as the acronym RSI, were John Mathews' invention, by his account a blend of the notions of repetitive movement injuries and stresses, and strains. Mathews said he was looking to make a link between poorly designed equipment or, worse, poorly designed work systems and their physical effects on those who had to operate them. He found Hunter's description of telegraphist's cramp in *The Diseases of Occupations* (1955) represented a powerful image of what could go wrong because of ignorance of the human effects of newly introduced equipment and work systems.

Mathews himself wrote the ACTU's *Guidelines*. He admitted that he drew heavily on documentary material, of which he received bundles, unsolicited, from people and organisations looking to influence the deliberations of the union movement. These published and unpublished articles on arm symptoms included material produced both in the Commonwealth Department of Health and in the NSW Department of Industrial Relations.

The ACTU's *Guidelines* provided 40 'further readings' and these references were extensively used by later medical writers on RSI. Mathews cited the apocryphal NHMRC *approved guide to prevention of repetition strain injuries* as the authority for the stand he was asking unions to take on preventive measures such as poor workplace design, tools and equipment and job design, workplace administrative procedures, and excessive work rates. He included Barbara McPhee's papers on prevention of repetition injuries as well as her citation base of Finnish and Japanese ergologists.

Mathews endorsed the work of Dr Jim Walker and the Workers' Health Centre at Lidcombe. He cited Walker's publication on tenosynovitis and the Centre's manual, *Occupational Over-Use Injuries: Information for Doctors and other Health Workers*, five of whose references entered his list of recommended further reading. He was particularly impressed with Walker's observation that carpal tunnel syndrome did not respond to surgery. He drew on Taylor's paper, *Repetition Injury in Process Workers*, and adopted nine of its references.

The ACTU's *Guidelines* also cited the publications of Cumpston, Ferguson and Elenor, along with media reports of the emerging epidemic and the Japanese epidemic of OCBD. It cited case reports of arm problems, including the occupation neuroses, which were referenced to the 1955 edition of Hunter's *The Diseases of Occupations*. Subsequent medical writers took up these recommended 'further readings' and added them to their reference bases.

Like Hunter, Mathews saw innocent workers as contracting physical injuries because they were being asked to work in the cold or to enter data at unrealistic rates. He saw them being designated either as malingerers or as needing surgical intervention. He believed that preventive remedies were obviously to hand. Mathews opted for the simplest remedy to curb the abuse at source: the redesign of work systems and keyboard work.

The union movement then engaged in a process of educating workers through its support of workshops, conferences, newsletters and audiovisual material, as well as circulating policy documents and submissions. Policy was formulated to slow down work that occupational health activists believed was being pushed dangerously fast. Calling for controls on the operation seemed to be a logical and sensible approach.

It was a source of satisfaction for Mathews to see the term 'RSI' and his reading list picked up in the medical literature, but this was followed by dismay as his intentions were distorted through litigation.

The notion of a repetitive strain injury and that it could be prevented by physical changes in the workplace was adopted and endorsed by various medical practitioners in late 1983 and early 1984, and several journal articles were published on the incidence and causes of RSI (Stone 1983; Browne et al. 1984; Ferguson 1984). Close examination reveals that some of the studies on which they had based their views were union-initiated surveys of workplace symptoms conducted during a period when arm symptoms were being targeted for attention, while their causes were being advertised, while anxiety was being generated about the dangers of work and while the reporting of symptoms was being rewarded with compensable sick leave and encouraged as a matter of policy.

THE AUSTRALIAN EPIDEMIC OF RSI

The 20 years after 1982 have been characterised by the belief that occupational tasks and conditions are capable of producing damage to the tissues in the arms. Medical legitimation has been available, as have certificates for time off work on compensation.

1982: *LASHFORD V PLESSEY*

On 25 March 1982, Justice Adrian Roden of the Supreme Court of New South Wales formally delivered judgment in *Lashford v Plessey*, the first successful common law claim for 'repetitive injury'. The case was backed by the AMWSU, acting for a woman engaged in the manufacture of domestic appliances.

Mrs Lashford was a 33-year-old married process worker who developed symptoms in 1978. Her work had involved placing pieces of metal and plastic strips into a machine. She claimed, through her examining doctors, to have suffered 'tenosynovitis', 'together with associated median nerve damage' producing 'carpal tunnel syndrome'.

Dr Browne gave evidence that she also suffered additional 'reflex sympathetic dystrophy syndrome superimposed on a severe occupational tenosynovitis'. Browne, who was later to publish on RSI in the *Medical Journal of Australia*, claimed that the plaintiff had suffered these injuries from having performed a task that involved repetitive movements.

Expert evidence was polarised between Dr Browne, a rheumatologist who claimed that Lashford suffered from four or five pathological conditions all of which were caused by her having worked repetitively, and Dr Bloch, a surgeon who claimed that the plaintiff showed 'no signs of teno-synovitis, epicondylitis, or any other itis' and that she was 'fit for full duties forthwith'.

The neurologist, Dr Ross Mellick, did not question the diagnosis of carpal tunnel syndrome and did not challenge electromyographic (EMG) findings. He saw no indication for operating, as he had experienced no surgical success with this condition. He also called it 'repetition injury'. The reliability of EMG studies was not questioned.

The evidence before the Court gave the judge the choice between believing that Mrs Lashford was injured by her work or that she was making it all up. No other formulation for her having such diffuse symptoms without clinical signs was offered. No psychiatrist was called. The symptoms described in the judgment and the multiplicity of diagnoses put forward suggest that Mrs Lashford's condition might have been diagnosed as somatization consequent on her well-documented psychosocial difficulties.

Awarding $72 000 (after deduction of workers' compensation already received by her), Justice Roden commented that medical testimony before the Court was contradictory and he complained of the difficulties of his task: 'The truth of the matter has to be that at least one of the doctors is completely and utterly wrong. It is obviously difficult for a person not qualified in the field of medicine to arrive at such a conclusion in respect of any of them.'

Having made this difficult and uncertain decision that the plaintiff had the injuries in this disputed situation, Justice Roden then had to decide on foreseeability and negligence.

Mr Osman, an employee of Plessey, had given evidence to the effect that some aspects of Mrs Lashford's task could have been replaced by machinery and the job could have been easier to perform. Justice Roden had also accepted evidence from Roy Pollock, the safety officer who had been a union delegate to the AMWSU for 14 years.

The judge nonetheless used judicial power to determine that 'repetition injury ... its aetiology and its mode of prevention were well known to the medical profession'. Moreover, he found that the disorder, repetition injury, was both known and preventable. He first found that there was a potential capability for eliminating some aspects of the task and, on that basis, he found that Plessey had been negligent. He reported that 'the existence of the risk should have been known to the defendants as it was well known to the medical and engineering professions and that, in fact, it was well known to the defendant through its own experience'.

The evidence before the Court was that the medical and surgical experts called by Plessey said, effectively, that they did not recognise any such syndrome in medical knowledge and they could not acknowledge the existence of such a condition in the claimant. The evidence had revealed that the condition, repetition injury, was known only to trade union delegates, workers and to the doctors who advised them. A generic disorder called repetition strain injury, or RSI, had not yet appeared in a refereed medical journal or a medical magazine. There had been no research demonstrating the allegedly traumatic aetiology of such a set of symptoms. That RSI was an injury was subsequently negated by its epidemic spread, but epidemiologists are rarely called as experts in Australian courts.

The case was argued in 1981 and the decision handed down in March 1982, that is, before any medical literature on repetition injury had been created at all. It was this legitimation that allowed the creation of medical literature. RSI was an example of a growing number of nomogenic diseases, those caused by the legal system.

Lashford v Plessey was not the first case legitimating vague and heavily contested subjective symptoms as evidence of compensable trauma. It was the first to adopt the term repetition injury and the first to deem it 'foreseeable'.

With the decision in *Lashford v Plessey*, the union movement had a judicially validated medical way of attributing symptoms to workplace injury. After this decision, there was legal precedent to enforce the removal of a complaining worker on pain of a successful common law claim for negligence. The employer now had a duty to warn workers of the risk of developing tenosynovitis or repetition injury, a duty that contained within it the very ideas that were to bring on an epidemic.

Following the success of *Lashford v Plessey*, many trade unions circulated guides to prevention and epidemics followed prevention campaigns. The epidemic peaked in Telecom and in the Australian Public Service in the December quarter of 1984 (see Figure 4.1) (Hocking 1986).

Figure 4.1
Telecom Australia RSI reports, 1981–86
SOURCE *Medical Journal of Australia*

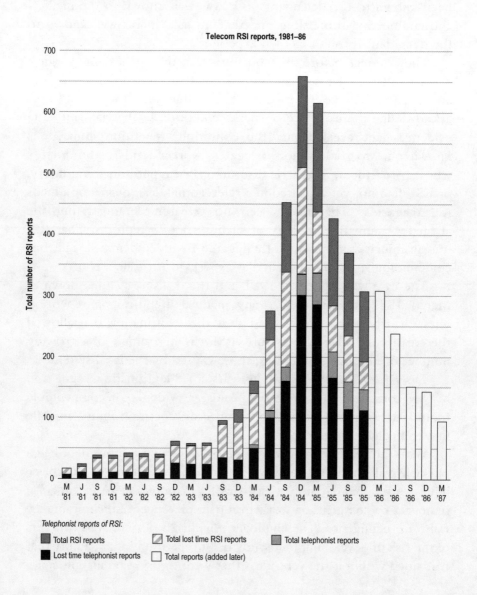

1982: PROMOTION OF DAMAGES
FOR TENOSYNOVITIS

Two barristers, Frank Stevens and Robert Dawson, promoted the decision in *Lashford v Plessey* in a pamphlet, *Damages for the Industrial Injury of Tenosynovitis*, which they published in 1982. The NSW Attorney General, Frank Walker, signalled the NSW Labor government's acquiescence to the idea when he launched it, saying:

> Repetition injury in process work has become one of the major industrial diseases plaguing the Australian work force. It currently accounts for over fifty percent of all applications for workers compensation by female employees and some 10% of male applications.
>
> Of recent date, however, in the Supreme Court of New South Wales, it was determined that such injuries give rise to damages in the tort of negligence. This fixes a new perspective into the field. Not only will the real economic cost of the injury be shared more evenly between employer and employee, the insurance industry will be called upon to carry an increasing burden of the cost.
>
> There are ways of avoiding injury through repetitive process work. These are clearly set out in the following publication. The penalties by way of damages for negligence in relation to the injury at work which will ensue if the advice is not taken, are also clearly spelt out.

Stevens and Dawson gave a dissertation on 'repetitive use syndrome', a legal construction of medical knowledge. Their view, defined in medical language, was that 'tenosynovitis was caused by the encrustation of the tendon sheaths by calcium, "capsulitis". Surgery, although frequently practised, is useless.' There was no cure for capsulitis.

In a comment on *Lashford v Plessey*, the authors predicted that, as more cases of tenosynovitis came before the courts, expert medical witnesses might, after the regular rejection of their evidence, become reticent to further damage their reputations by denying the presence of the disease.

The responsibility to defend claims against the NSW public service lay with the Government Insurance Office (GIO), which at that time was entirely state-owned. The NSW State Treasurer, Ken Booth, was persuaded to write to the general manager, Mr Bill Jocelyn, asking him not to use experts who would not acknowledge that RSI was an injury caused by work. Mr Jocelyn stood his ground. The state government, as its federal counterpart had done through its institutions, was prepared to throw away the defence of RSI cases in the interests of industrial harmony. This attitude was to cost the state dearly — the costs of the workers' compensation later had to be transferred to the state as they blew out by some two billion dollars by 2001. This blowout, attributed to lawyers, resulted in draconian legislation to limit payouts to the seriously injured along with everyone else. The opportunities for medico-industrial complex remained undiminished.

1983: THE FEDERAL LABOR GOVERNMENT

During 1981 and 1982, it had been a Liberal and National Coalition federal government that had conceded to the demands of the ACTU concerning management and prevention of RSI. In March 1983 a Labor government was elected on a platform of industrial reform. That year was the trough of a recession, the worst since the Depression of the 1930s. Australian Labor Party (ALP) policy included the restructuring of both industry and the public sector. Structural changes in employment were ongoing.

The Labor government was abandoning protective tariffs and, by 1985, many manufacturing industries were closing down, unable to continue without subsidy. New technology was being introduced at every level. Jobs were disappearing. There was a brief economic upturn, followed by another recession. By the end of the 1980s, around ten per cent of the workforce was unemployed and unemployment remained at more or less that level until 1992.

The Labor government's goals were economic stability and job creation. In February 1983 the ALP and the Australian Council of Trade Unions reached an historic agreement, the Accord, which was presented as 'a compact dedicated to economic growth and job formation'. Workers were to forgo pay rises to get inflation under control, and government would work on establishing industry policy, employment security and compulsory employer contributions to superannuation. After the signing of the Accord, union officials at every level transferred their attention to work conditions, health and safety issues.

In May 1983, nine months after publication of the ACTU's *Guidelines,* the Federal Executive of the ACTU adopted 'a health and safety policy' on the 'prevention of repetitive strain injury' and outlined a strategy to pursue 'through negotiation' with employers. The unions' negotiating currency was their ability to find those who had

RSI by early identification strategies and referral to doctors who would certify that they had this compensable disease.

The ACTU's *Guidelines* advocated early reporting of symptoms and ensured that workers were not victimised, that they did not experience financial loss because they complained and that they were transferred to non-repetitive work. Demands included detailed surveys to identify work areas and processes associated with them, encouragement of early reporting, education, and assurances that those who reported symptoms would be given rehabilitation, training, swift and full financial compensation and legal assistance in respect to claims at common law.

By 1983, RSI was the major issue for the clerical unions' health and safety campaign and the epidemic was approaching its peak.

1983: INTERIM NATIONAL OCCUPATIONAL HEALTH AND SAFETY COMMISSION: WORKSAFE AUSTRALIA

In May 1983, the federal government established the Interim National Occupational Health and Safety Commission (NOHSC), WorkSafe, locating it in Canberra with a budget of $12.1 million dollars for 1984 and a staff of 150, chaired by Dr Richie Gun. The ACTU had two representatives, including Ken Stone (no relation of Dr William Stone), who was at the time a junior vice-president and secretary of the Victorian Trades Hall Council and, in this capacity, the publisher of the *Health and Safety Bulletin* that had produced the ACTU's *Guidelines*. The Confederation of Australian Industry, the employers' representative body, had two members on the board and the state and federal governments had two representatives each. Three members were to be experts, of whom two were nominated by the Council of Occupational Health and Safety Professionals and one was co-opted by the Commission. These were experts in the sense of being medically qualified administrators, government employees, but not experts in the sense of being either trained or experienced in occupational health.

The Interim NOHSC and the NHMRC played a role in the creation of spurious medical knowledge and the legitimation of RSI. This was an example of a disease being created by powerful, authoritative, but non-scientific, authorities.

The NOHSC, which was increasingly called by its alternative name, WorkSafe Australia, joined the ACTU and together they set about improving occupational health by winning better working conditions for members.

The assertive policy of prevention was taken up and circulated by the ACTU to affiliated unions as well as by the Australian Public Service Association (APSA). An amalgamation had been arranged between the Australian Clerical Officers Association (ACOA) and the APSA. Policy for prevention was circulated and the reports of RSI started to rise everywhere. They were well documented in the Australian Public Service, (APS). Public servants were advised to seek union support as soon as symptoms developed.

As soon as symptoms develop ring the union.
Report them to the supervisor, first aid officer or nurse at work.
Ensure that the injury is noted in accident book.
Seek doctor's advice immediately.
Lodge a workers' compensation claim (form available from personnel section) with supporting medical certificates (keep copies of all documents).
If there are any difficulties in either completing the form or your superior officer accepting the claim form contact the PSA's welfare officer or women's industrial officer.
Your employer is obligated under the Workers' Compensation Act to lodge your claim within 7 days of receipt to the appropriate insurance company.
If after six weeks (minimum) there is no indication from the insurance company on the acceptance or rejection of your claim, contact the PSA. (RSI ACTU Policy. 1984.)

Support for RSI claims meant offering legal, medical and personal support for would-be claimants. Union officials vying for positions in the new amalgamated union made themselves conspicuously helpful in improving occupational health or winning better working conditions for members. Both of these noble goals were clearly announced in their respective policies.

The policy document included a definition of RSI, its causes and treatment and it reflected material which was to enter the *Medical Journal of Australia* a year or so later through a publication by Browne, Nolan and Faithfull.

Repetition strain injury and occupational over use injury are collective terms for a range of muscle and tendon injuries of the neck, shoulders, fingers, wrists, hands and elbows. Muscles and tendons are subject to two types of mechanical stress where (i) static loading or continuous contraction is required of the muscles of the neck, shoulder girdles and upper arms to support and fix the arm in a position of function. The arm may be regarded as a lever. (ii) dynamic loading repetitive movement is often required of the forearm, wrist, hand and fingers to execute a task.

Symptoms and their potential repercussions were described in this well-circulated policy document:

A repetition injury will usually show up as pain, swelling or numbness in, or around, the affected muscles or tendons. This usually occurs in the fingers, one or both hands, wrists and on arms. In some cases the shoulders, neck and or back muscles can be affected.

At first the pain, swelling or numbness may occur only occasionally while the repetitive movement is actually being done. However if preventive action is not taken the condition will worsen. It may then persist while the worker is doing non-repetitive movements or even when they are not using the injured area at all. Symptoms may worsen as the working day or week progresses.

In these documents, the ACTU and its affiliated unions described RSI as a progressive disorder that passed through five stages. Stage 1 involved symptoms of swelling and numbness, felt only at work and relieved on weekends. At stage 2, pain persisted overnight, with loss of ability to work. Stage 3 required job modification. Stage 4 lasted for months and was not relieved by rest. Stage 5 was the chronic and persistent condition of complete palsy, where the limb would have no functional use and the worker would never return to work.

The APSA had been concerned about the lack of career structures for DPOs and clerical assistants. These workers were largely women, and the underlying agenda was promoted as feminist. This initiative facilitated upward mobility for bright typists and DPOs and was a lasting success. Before this union push for workplace mobility for women, there was rarely a possibility for a bright keyboard worker or clerical assistant to transfer to an administrative position. During the epidemic, some were promoted while they had RSI and many completed degree courses on compensation payments.

The APSA insisted on controlling who were to be the agreed independent experts who were to conduct six-monthly monitoring of staff. The public sector unions negotiated a list of doctors who could be used by Commonwealth employers, so the outcome of a consultation on behalf of RSI could be predicted. The unions also encouraged complaints to various bodies about medical examiners who asked them questions about what they believed to be personal matters when the injury was in the arm.

In April 1984 a course was held on RSI to educate Commonwealth Medical Officers in work-caused paradigm of injury. These doctors, employed by the federal government, certified the condition and made recommendations concerning workplace changes. Commonwealth medical officers approved medical discharges from the APS. Early retirement on medical grounds was desirable, as medical discharge meant no loss of superannuation entitlements together with continuing payments of workers' compensation.

RSI first appeared in the Annual Report of the Commissioner for Compensation in 1985 as a reason for early medical retirement, and continued to appear, often 'with neurosis', until 1989, when whoever compiled those statistics stopped demarcating this cause of retirement from other medical conditions.

The Task Force into RSI in the APS documented the rise of RSI reporting during 1984 in the Commonwealth sector of employment (Figure 4.2).

Figure 4.2
RSI cases first reported in 1984

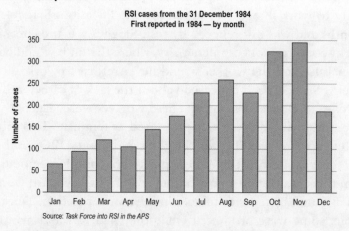

Source: Task Force into RSI in the APS

SOURCE Task Force into RSI in the Australian Public Service

5

RSI AND INSTITUTIONAL SUPPORT: MEDICINE AND GOVERNMENT

Show me a cultural relativist at thirty thousand feet and I'll
show you a hypocrite.

Richard Dawkins, *River out of Eden*

RSI was well established in the Australian Public Service before
December 1983, and it was well known in the trade union movement, to courts and to workers, yet no medical literature existed
about it in any professional medical journals. A traumatic disease,
created by judicial processes and previously unknown to medicine,
was visited on the medical community through the *Medical Journal
of Australia,* a refereed journal.

One could not call RSI a scientific fraud, because the process of
creating RSI was a process of social construction and, as such, it had
no relationship to science. A convenient fiction, a furphy, RSI was
created by trade unions' power, adopted by the National Health and
Medical Research Council, endorsed by Australian institutions, welcomed by government, and legitimated by publication in refereed
scientific journals.

Science was sacrificed to ideology as RSI suited political needs.
The epidemic highlighted the problematic nature of medical knowledge and it did so just as evidence-based medicine was to be promoted as an ideal.

The construction of RSI echoed an earlier scientific scandal.
Authority overran science when the Soviet government supported
Lysenko's idiosyncratic theories of plant breeding at the expense of
what was already known by geneticists who had won their knowledge

by conducting detailed and science-rich experiments, starting with Mendel, in the nineteenth century, who identified how traits were inherited. The Russian geneticist, Lysenko, rejected Mendel and the careful scientists who followed him in favour of a 'proletarian' approach to science in opposition to 'bourgeois' science (Joravsky 1970). Lysenko's methods produced crop failures in the Soviet Union and were responsible for the Chinese famine of 1958–62, the worst in human history, which caused the death of between 30 and 40 million people during the so-called Great Leap Forward. (Windschuttle 1999)

Joravsky coined a new term 'surrationalism', to describe the intellectual character of Lysenkoism. Jean Curthoys, writing about 'feminist science' (which she saw as a variant of junk science) later used the term 'surrational' to describe a situation where a 'show of rational discourse camouflaged an underlying refusal to meet the test of genuine reason'.

The thinking involved in RSI theory systematically failed to follow any logical approach. This lack of rationality was not conducive to the rational practice of medicine, nor was it compatible with it.

The RSI epidemic claimed victims. Thousands of trusting patients were given potentially dangerous medicines and unnecessary operations and they were disabled for long periods of time. Their families suffered. Their employers were penalised for doing harm, which, in fact, was done by the well-meaning institutions that peddled toxic beliefs that harmed. Some industries went bankrupt over massive insurance hikes.

Lysenkoism overran the courts as experts with demeanour presented opinions that had no scientific basis and impressed judges who felt that they were improving the world for workers. Members of the judiciary suspended their collective commonsense and joined the new social movement.

The kindest, most sympathetic physicians became vectors of a disabling illness, one caused by the ideas inherent in its name.

The NSW Workers' Compensation Commission's statistics suggested that there had been a tenfold increase in such claims between 1970 and 1985, subsumed under the labels 'synovitis', 'bursitis', 'tenosynovitis' and 'tendonitis'. In 1985 the new umbrella term for arm symptoms, RSI, accounted for more than 80 per cent of reported compensation claims for women Australia-wide.

Between August 1982 and June 1983, John Mathews' ideas were incorporated in the *ACTU Health and Safety Policy: Prevention of*

Repetitive Strain Injury (Mathews and Calabrese 1983) and into pamphlets and guides to diagnosis and prevention. Unions circulated these guides and pamphlets, and they found their way into many court reports. The epidemic was well under way. It was being documented in the Australian Public Service, by insurers and commissions and, in great detail, within Telecom Australia by the director of medical services, Bruce Hocking.

A new category of 'traumatic disease' appeared in compensation and medical retirement statistics (Commissioner for Employees' Compensation 1985–86).

By 1993, after new cases had slowed to a trickle, there were still well over a thousand employees receiving workers' compensation for RSI in the Commonwealth sector, which was serviced by its own legislation, Comcare. Much of the cost of the generous, perhaps extravagant, scheme was generated by the financial support, medical care and physical rehabilitation of cramp subjects who had been unable to return to their normal duties and had been maintained on compensation and in treatment for long periods.

When new cases started to decline, there was a steady increase in costs-per-claim as inventive, ineffective and poorly based remedies were billed to the insurer.

In late 1983 and early 1984, the *Medical Journal of Australia* introduced the acronym RSI and the concept of repetitive (and repetition) strain injuries through three papers. Their authors were Dr William Stone, a rehabilitation specialist practising in South Melbourne; Professor David Ferguson, an academic in occupational health; Dr Christopher Browne, a Sydney rheumatologist; Dr Bernie Nolan, employed in the NSW Department of Industrial Relations; and Dr Don Faithfull, a Sydney hand surgeon. All these doctors had already given expert evidence, advised government departments, sat on committees and addressed meetings. Their publications were very influential.

RSI reporting was rising fast. These publications let it be known that medical opinion, worthy of publication in a refereed journal, was available to support long-term invalidity and common law negligence cases. They were strongly criticised by Hadler as 'heuristic assertions and personal opinions'.

1983: DR WILLIAM STONE

In the first medical publication on repetitive strain injuries, Dr Stone's abstract informed the readership of the *Medical Journal of Australia* that the semi mechanized and repetitive nature of industry, the greater use of keyboards and the need to boost production during an economic recession had led to a huge increase in injuries.

Stone reported that the incidence of these syndromes was rising on account of technological change, increased rate of production and continuing ergonomic problems. His authority for this statement was the NHMRC *approved guide*.

Stone shared the terminology, *repetitive* strain injuries, a notion consistent with the viewpoint of John Mathews and the ACTU, whose *Guidelines* he cited in a later publication. The NHMRC *approved guide* shared this view but used a slightly different term: *repetition* strain injuries.

This article brought a new explanation for multi-local and non-recovering arm symptoms to a medical readership. As Stone's was the first article on RSI to be published in a refereed journal, when it was cited in the Index Medicus (Library of Congress Database, 1978–84) it created a completely new category, 'repetition strain disorders'.

Stone reported that he based his theories on his observations of patients complaining of arm symptoms in his rehabilitation centre in South Melbourne. He categorised 89 patients under the subheadings 'work' and 'road' and a further 100 by the acronym RSI.

In his article, Stone assumed a common, physical pathogenesis. Stating that it was his intention to clarify what he perceived as 'confusion of nomenclature', he introduced a classification of his own. Stone supported the 'incidence' of RSI by this same new nomenclature, using the patients who had been referred to him. His hypothesis was consistent with that of the ACTU and affiliated unions' policies. RSI was a new kind of injury and it had three main causes:

These are: (i) rapid, repetitive movements, as those of people operating keyboards; (ii) less frequent, more forceful movements, as seen in some assembly work; and (iii) static load, exposure to which is encountered in some areas of engineering, such as welding; the shoulder girdles of keyboard operators also experience static load. The term 'tenosynovitis' is particularly misleading, as very few repetitive strain injuries can be classed as purely, or even principally, tenosynovitis. Frequently, there is no component of tenosynovitis at all in these injuries.

The third category of cause, static load, referred to a situation where a worker had to maintain anti-gravity postures over prolonged periods. These activities were elevated to the status of causes of an injury. Stone reported that keyboard operators had RSI caused by the repetitive strain of keyboard work and that women had more of it than men did because women did more keyboard work.

In this report, the more common components of repetitive strain injuries were tendinitis, tenosynovitis, peritendinitis, tenovaginitis, myositis or repetition muscle injury, epicondylitis, chronic muscle strain, ganglions, and neuritis.

Stone added reflex sympathetic dystrophy (almost always after surgery) and thoracic outlet syndrome to that list. Both of these conditions had been hereto described as 'not RSI' in the Workers' Health Centre documents.

Stone said that he favoured the term 'occupational overuse injuries' but he did not explain how he differentiated the presumed aetiological factor, occupational overuse, from whatever was customary occupational or everyday use. His concept carried the implication that symptoms had been caused by physical entities, so they could be ministered with physical remedies.

Stone attributed the increase of RSI to the same external factors that John Mathews and the ACTU had chosen to target.

Stone's paper had 23 references. Ten comprised statistical information and press reports of the 1983 epidemic. He cited the NHMRC *approved guide,* which had used the term 'repetitive strain injuries' as well as the acronym RSI eighteen months earlier. Nine of Stone's references had been included in the recommended reading list appended to the ACTU's *Guidelines to prevention of repetition strain injury.* Other citations were the work of Ferguson and McPhee, a paper read by Nolan at a conference, the Japanese views of health hazards in elevated work rates and cash register operators during the Japanese Occupational Cervico-Brachial Disorder epidemic of the 1970s, a paper called Design and Disease, ergonomists, conference proceedings, and the 'prevalence of tenosynovitis and other injuries of the upper extremities in repetitive work' as well as the causes of tenosynovitis in industry.

The remaining three reference citations were of himself, an unidentified paper in *Occupational Health* on the incidence and remission rates of common rheumatic diseases, and a report on 'carpal tunnel syndrome and selected personal attributes'.

None of the cited papers gave any research support for the notion of the symptoms he reported being injuries caused by repetitive strain.

Stone's model of understanding of repetitive strain injuries was much the same as the model in the document that had become the NHMRC *approved guide*. This had been one of the source documents for the ACTU's *Guidelines*, which, together with the *approved guide*, had been the basis of the Administrative and Clerical Officers' Association policy on RSI and other union policy documents.

1984: PROFESSOR DAVID FERGUSON

Professor Ferguson's earlier work showed familiarity with the occupation neuroses, but that published after 1970 promoted a notion of a non-recovering tenosynovitis and, later, a generic RSI, attributed to poor posture and to those same work conditions the unions wanted to change. In 1984, he advanced a value-laden argument to the effect that a worker was entitled to have symptoms if he or she had worked under conditions that met his disapproval. Ferguson did not address causation. The notion that certain people were entitled to have RSI was to permeate the debate and litigation. Many claimants presented themselves to medical examiners and to others with an attitude of entitlement.

The increased use of safety officers created a demand for physicians in the new specialty of Occupational Medicine (Creighton 1982). Ferguson's academic department, the School of Occupational Health at the Commonwealth Institute of Health, was located on the campus of the University of Sydney. The injury model was taught there and, in later years, after Ferguson declared his change of mind, it was taught over his protests. Ferguson's early support had been pivotal in enabling the unions to use RSI in their industrial relations policy.

Ferguson's editorial, 'The "New" Industrial Epidemic' (1984), was the second and introduced the third of the 1983–84 publications on RSI in the *Medical Journal of Australia*. It gave RSI a certain academic respectability.

Ferguson commented on the Workers' Compensation Commission's rising numbers of soft tissue injuries. He did not reconsider the occupation neuroses. The epidemic spread of these conditions and their capacity to disable might have suggested that formulation.

Ferguson's editorial provided 21 references. Seven were to the group of himself, Stone, Browne, Nolan, Faithfull and McPhee. Five references cited his own work and one cited NSW Workers'

Compensation Commission statistics. Several were citations of ergonomists who, in turn, cited Stone and Ferguson in their publications. Ferguson cited Ramazzini (1700) (as did the ACTU's *Guidelines*), a condition with distinctive micro-pathology called *vilonodular tenosynovitis*, and eight papers on a variety of conditions, including rheumatism and the reliability of a vibration test in screening for predisposition to tenosynovitis.

None of Ferguson's cited papers referred to 'repetition strain injuries' except his, Stone's and McPhee's. Not one paper gave any pathological data to justify the use of the word 'injury' and none attempted to do anything other than to assume repetitive strain as a 'causal' entity.

In a *Medical Journal of Australia* editorial, 'Putting the Epidemic to Rest' (1987), Ferguson recanted, reporting that the very term RSI implied both injury and cause where neither existed. He had come to see the increase in RSI reporting as representing 'a remarkable psychosocial expansion of a long recognised and continuing occupational, medical and work design matter'.

1984: BROWNE, NOLAN AND FAITHFULL

In March 1984 another paper by a group of Sydney doctors, Browne, Nolan and Faithfull, 'Occupational repetition strain injuries: guidelines for diagnosis and management', appeared in the *Medical Journal of Australia*.

This article continued with the reasoning of its predecessors in that the only evidence of 'injury' was in the symptoms, which were wholly attributed to the 'injury'. Patients seen were apparently workers; hence the presumed injury was 'occupational'. Neither 'repetition' nor 'strain' was quantified; they were simply assumed.

RSI became a conglomerate of assumed occupational causes, diverse entities usually defined by specific local pathological changes, a hypothetical injury which was assumed to coexist with its manifestations as well as being the lesion responsible for pain, and weakness and fatigue of obscure origin.

Four new notions constituting a new disease entity were introduced in this paper. The first was that all conditions of traumatic origin in arms were manifestations of RSI. This confounded scientific study and collection of statistics. There was no symptom in the arm of a worker that could not be called RSI, as long as occupational causation was assumed.

The second notion was that RSI coexisted with a condition of traumatic origin. As such, RSI was responsible for clinical manifestations over and above such levels of pain and disability as could be reasonably attributed to a diagnosed lesion. A doctor could diagnose a condition of traumatic origin and could claim that the symptoms in excess of what he expected to see with this lesion were manifestations of RSI. This made RSI consistent with functional overlay or somatization, complicating injury.

The third new notion was that symptoms without signs were attributable to an injury that could arise at multiple sites. This allowed multiple-lesion diagnoses to be made if a doctor wanted to account for the abundant and scattered symptoms. This did not accord with any known traumatic disease in any Western diagnostic system, but was consistent with somatization suggesting injury.

The fourth idea introduced by the paper was that RSI was progressive. This idea passed for prevailing wisdom, was widely disseminated by well-intentioned laymen, and coerced physicians to protect the afflicted from further trauma. It had already provided the justification for Justice Roden's finding of negligence by Mrs Lashford's employer.

Browne et al. (1984) adopted the idea of 'stages I to III of RSI', a rhetoric which suggested that the extent of traumatic pathology could be deduced from the experience or behaviour of the sufferer. The authors denounced as 'incompetent' those 'personnel (medical and other)' who failed to make the diagnosis of RSI, warning that degeneration into 'advanced "RSI" and total invalidism' would be both inevitable and negligently caused if this were not done.

This paper provided 12 references, five of which were self- or perhaps group-referential in that two cited the NSW Workers' Compensation Commission, one cited a report of the epidemic in a lay newspaper, one cited Elenor, Dr Nolan's researcher at the NSW Department of Industrial relations, and one cited McPhee. Six cited various case reports of Pac-man phalanx, tennis elbow, arthritis and allied conditions, compression neuropathy and 'muscular metabolites with exhaustive static exercise of different duration'. None of the references provided contained empirical evidence to support the assertions in the paper.

The three papers published in the *Medical Journal of Australia* had a total of 55 references. More than 30 were either references to the group of authors' own work or to press reports of the epidemic.

The ergonomists and physiotherapists whose work was cited had cited the same group of doctors in a circular fashion. A few references were made to Japanese and Finnish statistics, both of which had been generated by polling questionnaires. The rest referred to case reports or familiar lesions.

1984: THE CAMPAIGN

On 28 September 1984, when the epidemic was at its peak, the Australian Public Service Association (APSA) launched a major national campaign on the issue of RSI in Australian government employment. The clerical unions had been circulating material promoting prevention since mid-1981, so to call this late operation 'the campaign' was something of an equivocation.

Rallies and marches coincided with the campaign opening by the secretary of the ACTU, Bill Kelty, who outlined, in heroic language, his perception of the situation facing younger workers and women workers generally who dealt with the new technology:

> RSI is the most significant health problem affecting APSA members and the union is taking a range of industrial and publicity action to stop this crippling work-related disease.

The campaign launch saw the official release of two publications, the APSA *RSI Sufferers' Handbook* and the *APSA RSI Policy*, together with brochures and posters that had been around for three years. The union claimed that there were already 3000 reported cases of RSI in the Australian Public Service (PSB Census 1986). In some areas, more than 40 per cent of keyboard workers were said to be affected.

The APSA described its submission as 'a vital component of the union's RSI campaign'. It referred to 'thousands of women employed in keyboard work, currently affected by this crippling disease' and the 'catastrophic effects of these injuries'. Kelty addressed 'particular areas in which government action is urgently required to reverse the current alarming situation'.

Two weeks later, John Dawkins, Minister for Finance and Minister assisting the Prime Minister on Public Service Matters, signalled the government's acceptance of the union's position. He acknowledged the anger and frustration of injured workers, emphasised their right to feel angry, and promised to address the problem.

1985: TASK FORCE ON RSI IN THE AUSTRALIAN PUBLIC SERVICE

The response of the federal government was to establish a task force 'to report to the government on the steps needed to be taken on the control, prevention and the management ... paying particular attention to the keyboard areas of employment'.

The Australian government's terms of reference were quite different from the considered response of the British government of 1911 when it called a departmental committee to discover the nature of telegraphists' cramp. Without understanding its nature, no one could prevent it. Prevention failed, as badly as killing sparrows might fail in preventing malaria and as badly as planting big potatoes failed to produce a decent crop in Lysenko's Russia. This failure wasted resources that could have been put to more useful purposes. Sick people did not get appropriate help with underlying problems and they submitted themselves to debilitating remedies.

The Task Force did not see itself as an inquiry into the nature and causes of RSI. It saw itself as a means of establishing employment standards for white-collar workers. It failed to understand the causes of RSI, yet it recommended expensive and useless, even counterproductive, procedures to prevent it. None of its recommendations was ever taken up. The Task Force recommended counting, documenting which sectors of the workforce were affected. This was to be done while symptoms and their causes were advertised and their reporting was encouraged as a matter of policy.

The Task Force muddied the waters by assembling medical information from diverse journals throughout the world about all the conditions that manifested in arms. Although it failed to differentiate the conditions of traumatic origin from those whose origin was psychogenic, it claimed that its evidence proved that RSI was not uniquely Australian.

Arm symptoms did occur all over the world, but the causal hypothesis of repetitive strain injury was uniquely Australian. Professor Ferguson claimed to have been the first to use a similar term. The NHMRC and John Mathews had first used and popularised the acronym. An inspection of Index Medicus would have revealed that Stone's paper in the *Medical Journal of Australia* (1983) had created the category.

A census of RSI cases found that the affected workers included an

air traffic controller, some computing staff, some librarians, a physiotherapist, a couple of reporters, a carpenter, a painter, some lines-
men, laundry assistants, cleaners, gardeners, labourers, technical
officers, graphic designers, draftsmen, meat inspectors, a parking
inspector, some motor mechanics, school assistants, dietitians, cooks,
nurses, kitchenmen, orderlies, tradesmen and one professor. This distribution of symptoms in the affected workforce undermined the
major causal hypotheses of rapid repetitive movements and overuse
and, to the critical observer, it disconnected any identifiable aspect of
the occupational task from the syndrome. However, the Task Force
ignored this dissonant evidence and its conclusions did not take its
implications into account.

Professor Nortin Hadler's meticulous critique of the concept was
written off with the ill-informed statement that 'Hadler has not done
any research'. My own submission was misquoted and misconstrued
beyond recognition.

The Task Force Report of 1985 did nothing to stem the flood of
cases. Unions all over the country made demands for extensive
changes in conditions of employment. In 1985 the *Journal of
Occupational Health and Safety* was launched. Its first issue was
entirely devoted to occupational stress and how it might be turned
from an industrial issue into a medical one. The second issue was
entirely devoted to the identification, prevention, management and
compensation of repetitive strain injuries. The journal continued to
publish papers in the injury paradigm right up to 1990. It reported
on legal successes and failures and encouraged publications that promoted interests associated with this emerging body of knowledge.

Trade unions would have thought they were well served by the
notion of occupational overuse syndrome (OOS), which allowed a
person to claim that overwork or some other aspect of a task had
caused an injury. Unions continued to control which experts could
used by the employer by the simple threat of calling work stoppages
if a worker was sent to a doctor who was not approved.

There was no shortage of workers prepared to become claimants.
Trade union journals and newsletters advertised the support that
could be made available to them from welfare officers, women's
industrial officers and volunteers. Volunteers, who in many cases
were women who had already successfully settled their own claims,
accompanied claimants to medical examinations. RSI support groups
and newsletters were given government grants (McIntosh 1986).

Certain doctors got referrals and favourable mentions in RSI group newsletters. Non-believers were spoken of in disparaging terms while unions attacked the integrity and income of those who spoke against the injury theory. Vilification extended to street demonstrations and insults. A system of complex rewards and punishments for doctors was established to ensure compliance with a changed set of social and gate keeping norms.

Union activists made efforts to exclude as medical assessors for insurers those practitioners who did not see RSI as an injury (*Canberra Times* 24 January 1986). Representations requesting that I be removed from the list of medical examiners for the GIO were made to the NSW Treasurer, who approached its general manger, Bill Jocelyn. Demonstrations were organised in two cities to attack non-compliant views and my presence (Bremer 1985; *Canberra News* 22 November 1985; *Courier-Mail* 27 July 1985; Douglas 1985; *Financial Review* 20 November 1985; ACTU 1986; *Canberra Times* 24 January 1986; *National Times* 17–23 January 1986).

Iain Ross, a lawyer then working as Occupational Health and Safety Officer for the Labor Council of New South Wales (the New South Wales equivalent of the Victorian Trades Hall Council; both are state branches of the Australian Council of Trade Unions) further criticised the GIO for using me as a medical assessor. The Labor Council pursued the matter further with the Minister and the Premier, the State Compensation Board, the Human Rights Commission and the Privacy Committee of New South Wales, and orchestrated a barrage of complaints to the Health Care Complaints Commission, all on the basis that my questions were 'offensive and irrelevant'. 'The injury is in the arm,' they complained, 'so why should she ask personal questions?'

Referred by word of mouth, workers reported symptoms at practices known for their sympathies. A footnote to Walker's paper in *New Doctor* in 1979 had noted: 'In the month since our survey was completed we have had 20 more new cases of tenosynovitis at the Workers' Health Centre. This is a further indication that the needs of sufferers of this condition are not being met by the usual medical and legal procedures' (Walker 1979). The pamphlet *They Used to Call it Process Workers' Arm* referred to 'uninformed and unsympathetic doctors' and invoked Walker, whose views had influenced this publication.

In 1984 Professor Nortin Hadler visited Australia under the auspices of World Health Organization in order to investigate the problem. He came at the invitation of the Commonwealth Department of

Health. A rheumatologist and epidemiologist of note and author of several textbooks on industrial medicine, Hadler had not seen a case of RSI before he came to Australia, but he had predicted that the politicisation of arm symptoms might occur, as had happened in the case of back pain in the 1930s (Hadler 1984). He attributed Australia's excess of symptoms to the great publicity given to the seriousness of the complaint, to features of the compensation system and to the manner of involvement of doctors and lawyers in the system. He said that he feared that a similar upsurge might happen with RSI in the United States and he was soon proved correct (Hadler 1986). The publication of Hadler's critique made little, if any, impact on the Australian Public Service, but it was the first substantial challenge to the injury paradigm.

The Task Force on RSI in the APS had failed, so a second inquiry was needed. The federal government took counsel from the newly formed National Occupational Health and Safety Commission, WorkSafe, which co-opted Dr Stone onto the Repetition Strain Injury Working Party.

In 1985 the Commonwealth Public Service Board issued a memorandum to all departments, adopting the Browne et al. (1984) view of RSI.

1985: WORKSAFE: NATIONAL OCCUPATIONAL HEALTH AND SAFETY COMMISSION

The Standards Development Standing Committee Working Party on RSI was set up with tripartite representation of employers, unions and states. It included Dr Bernard Nolan, Dr Bill Stone, Professor Ferguson and the ergonomist, Professor Stevenson.

The NOHSC produced an Interim Report (1985a). It was inevitable that it and its committees should adopt the same view of this epidemic disorder as the unions had done, as it employed the same doctors as consultants. On the one hand, trade union leaders had their network of legal and medical advisers, and on the other hand they had rank and file members influenced by alarming reports in the media.

Knowledge formation and legitimation had gone around in a circle. Medical specialists had been recommended by trade union interests to provide certificates for RSI subjects and to give expert evidence to courts. They were also chosen to provide expert advice to government and inquiries, and they now found themselves advising yet another government-initiated organisation. The fact that they held all these positions of influence further suggested that their views were legitimate.

The Interim Report was circulated and the NOHSC published a Model Code of Practice (1986). Like the Task Force, WorkSafe also claimed to have irrefutable evidence for an international experience of RSI with a history extending over several hundred years. In citing 60 papers on various arm disorders, the Interim Report expanded the Australian term RSI to cover all the arm symptoms and injuries about which it had been able to collect references and literature. Even scriveners' palsy from Shakespeare's time was renamed RSI.

The NOHSC went on to compile a set of recommendations on the prevention of what it characterised as an injury, conceding that it was perhaps exacerbated by emotional stress. How emotional stress was to exacerbate injury was neither explained nor elucidated, yet this idea also became common knowledge.

The Interim Report did made one significant policy shift in that it recommended that rehabilitation be undertaken in the workplace, putting an end to indefinite sick leave. Redeployment in a different, usually less repetitive, task was to be offered to the affected worker.

The recommendations of these two inquiries were read out to courtrooms as if they were expert evidence. Breaches of their code became grounds for suits at common law on the basis that negligence had occurred, most often in retrospective claims based on what the employer should have known. Thousands of claims were settled under state law and hundreds more were adjudicated by the Administrative Appeals Tribunal, which dealt with Commonwealth employees.

The lack of definition of RSI did not deter either the NHMRC or the NOHSC from giving out substantial funds for research within the occupational injury paradigm. Grants were made by NOHSC 'to establish a discrete medical diagnosis', 'to identify factors promoting progression of chronic pain to dependence and invalidism', 'to seek objective anomalies', 'to determine the role of the primary afferent pathway', 'to provide an early warning system for pre-clinical diagnosis of RSI', 'to assess thermography as a tool for diagnosis of RSI', 'to study the effects of sedentary activity', 'for an international comparison of keyboard work and the incidence of musculoskeletal problems', 'to investigate the health of working women',

'RSI in clothing trades', 'aetiological factors for RSI in musicians', 'to develop trade union strategies', 'to rehabilitate keyboard tele-phonists', 'to evaluate treatment regimes', 'to study compartment pressures', 'to study work practices', 'to screen information on RSI for the Special Broadcasting Service (SBS) in several community lan-guages', 'for ergonomic assessment of workplaces', and $39 000 was given to the Trade Union Medical Centre to 'provide a statistical pic-ture of 1000 RSI cases' which were to be seen, billed, and given mul-tiple diagnoses and multiple physical interventions there.

All these research grants were distributed to projects whose pro-tocols were within the dominant paradigm, which incorporated the assumption that the symptoms were the consequence of occupation-al conditions. No research was funded that was not based on the assumption of both occupational cause and physical injury. Nor was WorkSafe prepared to allow grant recipients the right to publish find-ings in journals of choice. It wished 'to receive data and then pub-lish, or not, as they judged appropriate'. One researcher sought to maintain his academic independence and returned such a grant, find-ing the conditions to be unacceptable (I. McCloskey, pers. com. 1993). None of these grants supported a re-evaluation of the causes of RSI. A number of proposals offering to do that were refused fund-ing. No results that questioned the 'caused by work' paradigm were published.

Dr Niki Ellis was made director of RSI National Strategy where she was responsible for promoting the prevention of RSI, euphemistically called 'preventive health services'. WorkSafe Australia published a dozen brochures, books, seminars and workshop pro-ceedings all under the umbrella of the RSI Information Service. No studies were funded by WorkSafe to correlate attribution theories with the incidence of reporting. No studies supported any correla-tion between the characteristics of the task and the development of the disorder.

AFTER THE AUSTRALIAN EXPERIENCE

The major textbook in the field of occupational health facilitated the transfer of RSI into the United Kingdom. In its seventh edition, *Hunter's Diseases of Occupations* abandoned its section on occupa-tional cramps and occupational neuroses and adopted the Australian view. Under multiple editorship, it produced a section called

Repeated Movements and Repeated Trauma. An admission of ignorance of the subject was followed by an outpouring of paraphrase of the Australian literature together with the reference base of the circularly self-referential Australians.

Supported by the writers' and telegraphists' cramp literature, RSI was given a history, an epidemiology, a pathophysiology and many remedies. Unenlightened about the different causes of neurosis and trauma, the authors stated: 'Occupational cramp may be considered a major variant of repetition strain injury'.

Epidemiology encompassed the Japanese OCBDs, the Australian statistics gathered on symptom reporting, the rise in incidence as measured by the NSW Workers' Compensation Commission, and the findings of WorkSafe. The section on aetiology was the same as that adopted by the NHMRC and documented by Stone, Ferguson, Browne, Nolan and Faithfull.

On the issue of cause, the authors cited the so-called internal document compiled by the non-medical researcher in the NSW Department of Industrial Relations, Elenor. His qualifications for putting together a report about medical matters suitable to be cited in a medical textbook were never revealed and his paper has remained unavailable to me and to outside researchers.

In the section on pathophysiology, the authors acknowledged the absence of an inflammatory process, but they put forward an entirely new hypothesis concerning 'the impairment of blood flow leading to delayed clearance of metabolites and thereby to muscle fatigue'. No study was cited to support the notion that blood flow was actually impaired.

According to the authors, diagnosis was to be made through taking a thorough occupational and clinical history, which collated contextual and circumstantial evidence.

Hunter's Diseases of Occupations advised the doctor to take a detailed occupational history to establish that the worker had been engaged in previous occupations involving repetitive duties. Doctors were advised to pay attention to previous symptoms of RSI (presumably as the patient recalled them when their existence was suggested), to the anatomical pattern of symptom evolution, to the delay before advice was sought and action taken, to the relationship between work schedules and symptoms and to (assumed) precipitating factors such as overtime bonus incentives, increased work rate, recent return from pregnancy or vacation. This was taken from the ACTU's *Guidelines*.

The authors also adopted the notion that RSI could coexist with other syndromes of constitutional origin, such as arthritis and cervical spondylosis, then recommended a number of expensive investigations which could be undertaken, including laboratory, radiological, electromyographic and thermographic investigations and the use of an 'isokinetic dynamographer'. They did not specify what benefit might accrue to the worker or to her employer from any of these investigations.

No rationale was offered for how these rituals might elucidate the subject, or what results might be achieved by all or any one of them. The section on treatment recommended all the remedies that had been reported as unsuccessful in previous editions of this same textbook.

After publication of the 1987 edition, specialists involved in the defence of RSI claims lobbied the editors. The book's version of causation was deconstructed in these submissions. When they were approached about the origins and reliability of this material, the publishers expressed concern and referred the matter back to the editors. No more was heard. In some jurisdictions, this publication might be at risk of legal action for providing careless advice that was productive of misdiagnosis and disability.

The next edition of this influential textbook was published in 1994. It acknowledged the existence of a controversy about the origins of these disorders but again based its text and references on the work of the Australians.

THE SPREAD OF RSI

RSI spread to New Zealand, then to the United Kingdom, Canada and the United States. The first cases in the United Kingdom were reported in the popular press with claimants posing with their arms in splints. Brian Pearce analysed the British press coverage of RSI in his dissertation on the epidemic as moral panic (pers. com. 1997). The first claims involved keyboard users in October 1991, and were won by the plaintiffs, inspiring headlines including 'RSI victory threatens flood of cases' in *The Times* and 'Keyboard injury awards may lead to thousands of claims' in the *Daily Telegraph*. The claim in *Mughal v Reuters* in 1993 was successfully defended and reported as a test case, but it was by no means the first by a keyboard user to reach the High Court.

In September 1994 the British Trade Union Congress (TUC) claimed that RSI was costing UK industry £400 million a year. Owen Tudor of the TUC's *Don't Suffer in Silence* campaign called for urgent action from the Health Department. He was quoted in the most prestigious scientific journal in the world, *Nature*, as saying: 'With two hundred thousand sufferers a year, the Health Department should set up a whole research program' (Verral 1994). *Nature* declined to publish my 300-word critique of the TUC position. By early 1995 there were calls for a governmental inquiry into RSI. It was said on BBC TV (11 January 1995) that there were 200 people involved in litigation, but there were many more than that.

The notion of cumulative trauma was formally transferred to the United States in 1986 when the Association of Schools of Public Health together with the National Institute of Occupational Safety and Health proposed 'national strategies for the prevention of leading work-related diseases and injuries'. Cumulative trauma disorders were not entirely new — they had been promoted by a small number of physicians and surgeons for many years before this happened (*Financial Review* 4 March 1986).

This public health initiative was followed by an epidemic of claims. In Utah, Arizona and Colorado keyboard telephonists who performed several hundred keystrokes an hour (three or four words a minute) reported symptoms and attracted the attention of surgeons rather than physicians. In Denver the 30 directory assistance operators who sued the manufacturers of keyboards had been subjected to a total of 70 invasive surgical procedures for entrapment neuropathies, reflex sympathetic dystrophy, thoracic outlet syndrome and tendon separation, ganglions and scar revisions. Only nine were spared surgery. This meant that there were more than three interventions on each telephonist, with operations done on different parts of the arm, each with a different rationale (Hadler 1992).

A surgeon reported on a meat packing plant in Illinois, where she noted an increase from two to 58 hand operations between 1971 and 1983 (Masear 1986a, 1986b). Masear's criteria for surgical intervention were symptoms involving two radial digits and she resisted any suggestion that her patients were afflicted in an epidemic of occupational cramp or neurosis.

6

THE EXTENT OF
THE AUSTRALIAN EPIDEMIC

A fashion is nothing but an induced epidemic.

George Bernard Shaw

THE CREATION OF
STATISTICAL DATA

The only inference that can safely be drawn from all the available information is that there was an epidemic of medically certified work disability on account of arm symptoms.

This disability was indifferently attributed to conditions collectively known as RSI, in sectors of the workforce where claims had previously been rare. Tenosynovitis, previously known only in workers whose tasks involved twisting movements, suddenly afflicted the keyboard trades. 'Functional overlay' and 'functional disorder' no longer featured in medicolegal reports, nor did occupational cramps and neuroses. Inflammatory conditions whose known natural history normally spanned days or weeks were persisting for months and years.

Statistics were collected by different agencies, by various methods, using diverse criteria in disparate regions. In New South Wales there was an 11-fold increase in claims for arm problems between 1970 and 1985, from 600 to 6948. Between 1979 and 1980 absenteeism attributed to these disorders doubled and between 1980 and 1982 it trebled (NSW Workers' Compensation Commission). In 1986 the Commission stopped collating these overview statistics.

CHANGES IN LEGISLATION

The ACTU had long been lobbying for occupational health and safety legislation and the state governments duly legislated for standards in accordance with the Williams Report.

Entrepreneurial enterprises took advantage of these opportunities to provide services to injured workers. RSI subjects were their most numerous clients and they soon outnumbered those injured by cars and in industrial accidents. The recruitment of medical and paramedical personnel to workplaces that had formerly functioned without them became a costly exercise. As far as sufferers were concerned, treatment was of no use at all, but costs rose continually as increasingly elaborate investigations and remedies were billed to the insurer.

Morbidity and disability attributed to soft tissue injuries undid the gains made in other areas of occupational health. The major issue was not the increase in number, as claims fell in other areas, but the rising cost per claim. Medical costs of RSI undid any gains made from the reduction of industrial accidents (NSW Workers' Compensation Commission, Annual Reports, 1970–85).

In 1984, 2263 people in New South Wales were said to be involved in compensation for RSI (*Sunday Mail* 2 December 1984) and by 1986, 80 per cent of the new claims were made by women, for arm problems.

Accident claims peaked in New South Wales in 1981–82, with more than 145 000. Then, including the RSI epidemic, total workers' compensation claims fell by about 30 000 cases between 1982 and 1983 and this drop was sustained. However, the fall was not the consequence of an Occupational Health and Safety (OHS) initiative, as it anticipated the *Occupational Health and Safety Act* by a year or more. Rather, it reflected increasing unemployment and a shrinking workforce.

It took longer for the real gains of OHS legislation to come through, and real gains were indeed made and sustained by effecting changes to manual handling and construction processes. Limits to lifting and other simple regulations had hugely beneficial effects on the injury rates in heavy and construction industries.

The efficacy of remedial services was never assessed. Injury managers in insurance offices complained of medical practices that seemed to be costly black holes, but they had to pay up. Claimants complained that treatments did not help, but complied to prove that they were sick.

Group demands were quickly met in the public sector and

WorkSafe Australia slowed down its proselytising. Manufacturing industry could do little other than remove unskilled process workers from their production line and manufacturing tasks, which had come to be seen as harmful.

Insurance premiums rocketed. In one commonly cited example, a manufacturing company employing 150 people had its premium increased from $50 000 to $150 000 in one year, because three RSI claims had been made against it. Some enterprises closed (Dressing 1981). Employers continued to protest (Gittins 1986). The rising costs reflected upon the activities of the unions, which, supported by WorkSafe Australia, promoted symptom discovery by untrained personnel.

Australian law took an agnostic view of opinion evidence. No opinion was considered out of order and no treatment was inappropriate if it had been ordered by a doctor. This absence of restraint encouraged physicians to undertake experimental investigations and remedies and courts declined to curb such practices. WorkSafe organised conferences to provide a showcase for the proponents of the injury theory, whom it openly favoured, to present their research. It paid airfares and hotel costs. I was formally invited to observe one in Sydney, but I was never invited to speak.

Against this background, extensive changes were made in federal and state compensation legislation. The legislators abolished payment for symptoms without signs as if they had intuitively differentiated disease states from other conditions. In 2001, and, again, in 2002, a completely new system of workers' compensation was introduced, one that gave very little to the injured worker. It was intended to exclude lawyers and courts, but the new scheme continued to support the medico-industrial complex, putting doctors rather than lawyers on tribunals.

THE RISE OF RSI IN NEW SOUTH WALES AND OTHER STATES

No region was spared the epidemic. Attributions varied with the pet theories of regional experts. South Australia used a unique type of accident code for injuries whose cause was seen as repetitive movement. Insurers indicated that this group has been classified by location: 'upper limb', 'back' or 'other'. The picture that emerged, according to Dr Richie Gun, was not so much of an epidemic as an endemic group of conditions that remained as the epidemic faded.

The figures from South Australia did not show an increase in time lost from work similar to that in other states. The clinical experience of Dr Mark Awerbuch, who saw hundreds of cases in Adelaide, suggests that the RSI epidemic was simply not recorded in the state's official statistics (Awerbuch 1984, 1985).

Low incidence rates in professional, technical and executive occupations suggested, to those inclined to see workplace causes, that job dissatisfaction was important in the causation of RSI. However, no study confirmed that hypothesis and many claimants in ordinary jobs insisted that they were satisfied with them.

COMMONWEALTH SECTOR

The first sector exposed to preventive measures was the Australian Public Service, which commissioned the Task Force on RSI in the APS to record its incidence. At the end of 1984 there were 3103 sufferers. This increased by more than 600 cases a quarter to a cumulative total of 6825 reports, reached at the end of 1985. There were more than 1000 separations, these being medical retirements and failures by probationary staff to become permanent in the five quarters from March 1986.

Common law claims for RSI increased by 86 per cent. Costs of RSI in the APS in the December quarter of 1985 alone came to $9.5 million and only sporadic information was available about all this.

After 1990, Comcare became the agency responsible for the rehabilitation of injured people in the Commonwealth sector. Available statistics indicate that the number of new cases fell after 1985 but rose again in 1991. In fiscal 1996, 25 per cent of all claims received were for upper limb problems or attributed to body stress, while 17 per cent were stress claims. RSI continued to flourish in the Commonwealth sector of employment largely because of the administrative arrangements in Comcare for managing the claims. Strains excluding the back consistently accounted for more than 30 per cent of the total, or 4682 claims out of 15 813 (Comcare 1995–96). Occupational Overuse Syndrome claims numbered 1474, or seven per cent of the total. The average cost per claim was $15 191.

TELECOM AUSTRALIA

In the late 1970s and the early 1980s a new technology, which bypassed operators, was being introduced into Telecom Australia.

Although management reassured employees that there were to be no retrenchments, both job value and security were at issue and union activity increased. Voice-operated equipment further reduced the value of the work and the diminishing workforce was encouraged by its union to see the physical component of being a telephonist as stressful. From the late 1970s, pamphlets and fliers concerning RSI and how it should be dealt with were circulated extensively within Telecom. Although working as a keyboard telephonist rarely involved more than 400 keystrokes an hour, thousands of telephonists developed RSI from keyboard work, both in Australia and overseas. Doctors did not know what they were talking about when they certified hundreds of keyboard telephonists as having RSI or overuse syndrome from keyboard work, a rate equivalent of typing a couple of words a minute.

Over a period of five years, the direct cost of the epidemic to Telecom was $15 million.

THE DECLINE OF THE EPIDEMIC

Unions eventually stopped their prevention campaigns and the epidemic, which had followed them, ran out of steam. Authoritative non-victims speculatively attributed it to changes in the perception of RSI. The Australian Medical Association, the Hand Club representing hand surgeons, and the Royal Australian College of Physicians criticised the concept and called for a new name, not knowing that one was already available.

A conference called *Medical Mythology* was held in Sydney in November 1985 to deliver the view that RSI was epidemic occupational cramp. It attracted union-organised demonstrations: banner-carrying women in splints blocked city streets in Sydney and, later, in Brisbane. The material that attracted this furore was my paper, *Neurosis in the Workplace*, which was still being held up by the referees of the *Medical Journal of Australia*. Increasing awareness of the emotional origins of arm symptoms made them less attractive to report. It might also have been that those who were vulnerable to the temptation to adopt sick role behaviour on the basis of RSI had all already done so.

In an editorial in the *Medical Journal of Australia* (1987), called 'RSI: Putting the Epidemic to Rest', Ferguson resiled from his earlier position. Having earlier believed that RSI implied both injury and cause where neither existed, he had come to see the increase in RSI reporting as representing 'a remarkable psychosocial expansion of a long recognised and continuing occupational, medical and work design matter'.

In the same issue Dr Leslie Cleland published a paper called '"RSI" A Model of Social Iatrogenesis'. Citing Ivan Illich, he warned against social iatrogenesis, iatrogenesis by nomenclature and the effects of the compensation, of the rehabilitation system, of system dysfunction and of the potentially adverse effects of incorrect labelling, 'including wasteful ill-directed research in that data gathering without rigorous testing of hypotheses [which] served the entrenched opinions of pseudo-investigators without adding usefully to scientific knowledge'. Cleland described how the prospects of a settlement fed an industry of futile professional activity, which sometimes rendered the victim beyond rehabilitation. He pointed out that this epidemic of illness bore out the claim that medicine, as suggested by Illich, was a disabling profession. Dr Graham Wright also reported that the RSI concept had failed (Wright 1987).

Dr Bruce Hocking, Director of Medical Services for Telecom Australia, published research based on surveys and employment data, which ensured the ultimate failure of the notion of an occupational overuse syndrome. Allowing for differences in interpretation of symptoms and the variable nomenclature, Hocking published in graphic form a table of the rise of total reports, telephonist reports and lost time.

The inverse relationship between the number of keystrokes involved in a task and that sector's predisposition to RSI was revealed in a detailed analysis of which sector, in Telecom, was claiming to suffer from it.

Hocking's findings showed that their population of typists and computer operators who performed 12 000 or more keystrokes per hour provided only 17 reports, a rate of 34 per 1000 workers. The clerks with mixed duties, typing, data processing and other keyboard activities provided 1421 cases, a rate of 284 per 1000 workers. Telephonists whose jobs entailed, on an average, a dozen keystrokes for each call or about 400 keystrokes an hour provided both the greatest number of cases (1886) and the highest rate (343 reports per 1000 workers). These figures reflected the findings of the Departmental Committee into Telegraphists' Cramp in 1911, which had found that the fastest and busiest operators, night-shift telegraphists who had done the most work, reported no cases.

There were marked differences in incidence between telephone exchanges between states and within states.

Hocking also reported that 83 per cent of sufferers were female, with younger age groups over-represented in female but not in male workers. There was no relationship between the duration of employment and the incidence of symptoms. The condition was both more frequent and more severe in part-time telephonists. There was no increase with increasing age. The higher rate in part-time workers further failed to support a relationship between the duration and extent of equipment use and symptoms. Supervisory style was not found to be an important variable.

There was no identifiable relationship between the development of RSI and technology, and none at all with the ergonomics of the workstation. A cluster of cases had occurred around 50-year-old magneto equipment while, at the same time, many workers blamed modern technology. Non-work stress, such as family strife, was an important variable but no details of these more personal findings could be given.

Of Telecom employees who reported symptoms at the height of the epidemic, 16 per cent went on to take long-term leave on compensation and had to be medically retired. This highlighted the serious failures of treatment and rehabilitation. Some of the affected telephonists were later rehabilitated for work by being given voice-controlled computers and some developed difficulties with their voices.

The marked differences in cost per case between states reflected different approaches to case management, a feature which, Hocking observed, was not appreciated in WorkSafe management guidelines. Hocking reported that rehabilitation was costly and that it resulted in losses to Telecom. Hocking also reported that the decline in the epidemic of OCBD in Nippon Telephone and Telegraph had been attributed to the introduction of lightweight headsets, but these had already been in use in Australia when the epidemic started. Hocking suspected this measure only had a placebo effect.

The 1987 issue of the *Medical Journal of Australia* did nothing at all to help those already afflicted. Common law cases were won and lost. A high profile case, *Cooper v Commonwealth of Australia*, was lost in front of a jury in the Supreme Court of Victoria in 1987, in spite of Professor Ferguson referring to Cooper's work environment as 'terrible'.

CONCLUSION FROM THE EPIDEMIC SPREAD

The sudden rise in the numbers of RSI case reports was not consistent with the notion that RSI was an injury caused by repetitive strain. Nor was its distribution in the workforce. No workplace factors emerged as an overriding cause for cases. RSI was better explained by the notion that it was caused by the preventive strategies that promoted beliefs and provided opportunities for action. This epidemiology provided further support for the notion that RSI was an epidemic of hysteria or somatization, while its context confirmed that it was caused by unverified beliefs, that combined with the knowledge that attendance on certain medical practitioners would have certain consequences.

The fact that repetitive strain and injury had been soundly falsified did not prevent other countries from passing legislation within the injury paradigm. In March 1999 the Federal Occupational Safety and Health Administration in the United States issued draft ergonomic standards to address repetitive strain injuries and other repetitive motion injuries.

7

SOMATIZATION IN THE FORM
OF WRITERS' CRAMP

HOW DO PHYSICIANS
RECOGNISE SOMATIZATION?

The charge most commonly levelled by patients and health workers against doctors who diagnose somatization is that this dismisses the patient's complaint as somehow not 'real' or even as 'imagined' (Murphy 1989). However, although they are caused by ideas and emotional factors, the pain, symptoms and disabilities of hysteria and somatization are as real as any others.

Speaking on Radio National's *Occam's Razor* in 1986, Dr Nick Crofts said:

> I understand that there are psychiatrists in existence today who consider that RSI is a form of 'hysterical conversion disorder'. I hope you have noted the quotation marks, because I consider that such terms say a lot more about the person who uses them and nothing about the person they are used against.

Crofts displayed the attitudes adopted by the doctors who had become involved in the diagnosis and treatment of RSI. He took the position that psychosomatic meant imaginary, all in the head, and that such a diagnosis was used against a patient.

Normally, a patient who has experienced a symptom is relieved to learn that he or she does not have a disease. One would expect a man to be relieved to know that his chest pain signalled emotional distress rather than myocardial infarction, or a woman to know that her symptom was cramp, not a potentially crippling injury. However, the evidence suggests that there is another population, one that seeks out doctors who are prepared to give them a gloomy prognosis that confirms the beliefs they wish to have about their bodies, that they are indeed injured. Furthermore, this population not only seeks out, but also stays with, doctors who cannot help them recover.

Dr Crofts admonished patients to ask their doctor: 'How do you know?' And it is fair enough for patients to demand justification of a diagnosis. Doctors should be able to explain why they consider a given set of symptoms to be psychogenic.

Somatization is not a diagnosis to be made solely by exclusion. Somatization can also be a positive diagnosis that requires the presence of several criteria. Symptoms suggest a disease or injury in the body (hence, the term somatoform) and are not fully explained by a medical diagnosis. The patient is experiencing a stress that can be relieved or a conflict that can be resolved by the development of the symptom. In practice, a somatizing patient will have concurrent sensory and motor symptoms of a kind that occur together only in rare neurological conditions, which all have overt clinical signs. The patient has a firm idea of what is wrong and vigorously defends herself against advice to the contrary. Impairment is greater than warranted by symptoms, which move from place to place and cannot be explained by one, two or three pathologies and have not responded to the treatments for the conditions they suggest or mimic.

DIFFERENTIATING CRAMP FROM DISEASE

Diseases have specific criteria and their characteristics have been the subject of many textbooks. Such complaints as constitute somatization in upper limbs need to be distinguished from diseases that they suggest or mimic. Functional disorder in the form of cramp can mimic disease, may coexist with disease and may prolong symptoms from old lesions well past their expected recovery time.

The examination of the medical file of a cramp subject reveals how changing symptoms attract multiple diagnostic formulations over the period of the affliction. As Hércule Poirot might say: 'There are too many clues'.

DIFFERENTIATING CRAMP
FROM DISEASES OF NERVES

Cramp symptoms move from site to site and suggest concurrent involvement of the sensory and motor nervous systems. Doctors recognise conversion or somatization symptoms when they are of a classical glove-and-stocking or long-glove distribution. Glove distribution is the traditional format of hysterical symptoms because it is determined by the idea of a hand yet does not accord with its nerve supply. Similarly, somatoform symptoms occur on the left side of the chest, corresponding with the location of the heart, whereas angina is experienced in the middle of the chest and in the neck or arm.

During the RSI epidemic, ulnar neuropathy and carpal tunnel syndrome (CTS) were often diagnosed, but surgical treatment was never successful. The diagnosis of CTS cannot be made by abnormal electrical conduction studies alone. If symptoms and signs are limited to the distribution of the median nerve distal to the place in the wrist where it passes through the carpal tunnel, they always respond to carpal tunnel release.

EMG studies are said to show 'impaired median nerve conduction, carpal tunnel syndrome'. Such tests are generally considered so unreliable as to be useless, as 40 per cent of asymptomatic people older than 40 have slow nerves and no symptoms at all (Toyonaga et al. 1978; Nathan & Doyle 1988). Unless symptoms involve the exact territories of the suspect nerves, no more and no less, then surgical intervention will be unsuccessful, no matter what nerve conduction studies indicate. Release of the nerves for any other problem is unsuccessful and, after initial respite, symptoms recur in greater profusion. The clinician who has originally failed to recognise a functional disorder then falls back on a diagnosis of functional overlay.

Peripheral neuritis involves the feet long before the hands and there is generally an overriding medical reason for having it. A neurological examination of a cramp subject would reveal that all the relevant muscles and peripheral nerves are intact and that there is no muscle wasting. Atrophy in splinted or over-rested limbs is common and affects all muscles. In contradistinction to cases with neurological lesions, wasting of specific muscles does not occur in cramp subjects.

Attributing cramp symptoms to radicular irritation at the cervical spine is a neurologically unsound formulation. When nerves come out of the spinal column, they mix with each other and then go to a recognised distribution, so vague pains cannot properly be attributed to them. Such a diagnosis rests on signs that should relate specific muscle weakness to discrete sensory deficits, and these are not found. The resemblance ends if the motor deficits expected to occur with the suspected lesion cannot be found.

DIFFERENTIATING CRAMP
FROM TENOSYNOVITIS

The contention that keyboard work predisposes to tenosynovitis is anecdotal, not expert. Stenosing tenosynovitis is not a reported disorder of typists, yet writers' cramp, in a painful mode, has recurrently and erroneously been attributed to tenosynovitis. In 1986, a search using the Medline database found that occupational cramp alone was associated with typists. The more recent confusion, occasioned by misinformation, has spawned a huge number of reports involving the near-enough diagnosis of endless afflictions and this can be confirmed by serial searching the literature five years at a time.

Cramp is differentiated from tenosynovitis primarily by its excessive symptomatology in both motor and sensory modalities and secondarily by its failure to recover with the usual treatments for inflammation or injury.

De Quervain's tenosynovitis is a specifically located lesion. It causes localised pain and sometimes stenosis and it is easily and quickly cured by surgery. However, cramp symptoms do not respond, and de Quervain's syndrome that persists after surgery is called 'intersection syndrome', to account for persistent pain (Reagan 1985).

DIFFERENTIATING CRAMP
FROM DISEASE OF MUSCLES

The suggestion that cramp is a disease of muscles is not corroborated by any reliable relationship of tissues used to occupational tasks. Moreover, there is no known organic disorder in which a group of muscles becomes dysfunctional and painful for one intentional activity but not for another.

The idea that RSI is a musculotendinous injury fails to account for multiple sensory symptoms and for generalised weakness and fatigue in many subjects. No disorder is known in which collapse, exhaustion and pain follow activity, sometimes hours, sometimes a day or two later.

DIFFERENTIATING CRAMP
FROM MYOFASCIAL DYSFUNCTIONS

One cannot assume that pseudo-neurological symptoms, which are not caused by peripheral neuropathies, are functional in origin. Tingling in fingers might also be a referred symptom from strained or pulled forearm muscles; it is experienced along the finger that the traumatised muscle supplies (Travell & Simons 1983).

Myofascial dysfunctions, cramps, spasms and occupational myalgias are all task-related and, like their counterparts in sport, they go on to a normal, predictable recovery with rest or treatment. Diagnosis of such lesions lies in the ability to correlate muscles affected with muscles used. Testing muscles in functional groups identifies the tasks and actions that have made those muscles sore, especially at their insertions, as with epicondylitis. The action that caused the dysfunction is the one that elicits the pain.

Carrying shopping bags or a briefcase on part of the hand commonly causes soreness in forearm muscles supplying the flexors of the middle, ring and little fingers. This can last for months, especially if it is aggravated, but it is not a result of an occupational task, that has not involved that activity. Arthritis in various locations is not a mobile symptom and there are biological and radiological signs of it.

DIFFERENTIATING CRAMP FROM OVERUSE AND MISUSE

Overuse syndromes are a matter of common knowledge, particularly in limbs unaccustomed to activity. Physical injuries start to recover when put to rest and run a predictable course. Somatization endures beyond these time limits and has an entirely different natural history.

OCCUPATIONAL MYALGIAS

A task might excite symptoms that develop so quickly that it cannot be fatigue. This is called 'intention myalgia' and, as far as I can see, it is reported only during epidemics. The symptoms coincide with a belief that the task is intrinsically dangerous. Persistent myalgia afflicts people who are tense or angry, want to be somewhere else and are obliged to work. Their emotions are not necessarily related to issues in the workplace. Their problems, like those of school-phobic children, probably originate at home. Farmer (1986) construed tension or intention myalgia as a signal from the body suggesting, 'Perhaps your body is telling you that you don't want to be at work?' Myalgia, extending to normal domestic chores, invites us into the literature of chronic pain and fibromyalgia, conditions which, like RSI, can more reliably be related to the beliefs of doctors and to predicaments of the patients and than to pathology in the body.

DISTURBANCES OF SENSATION

Neuralgic, stabbing, shooting, sharp or dull pain, burning, numbness, pins and needles, hot and cold and cramping are all reported affecting multiple sites, crossing into the unused limb and spreading in any direction from their origin.

A subjective sensation of being swollen was a common complaint, but swelling was not visible. Unaware that the dominant hand is larger than the other, some claimants present this as proof of abnormality. Symptoms came in various combinations and changed frequently in response to suggestion. Some claimants seemed to be fascinated with the details of their unusual sensations. Glove distribution affected the most guileless subjects. Other locations accorded with the body part the claimant perceived as 'overused'. A random sensation might be inaccurately remembered.

Reports reflected information available in pamphlets, symptom lists and guides to diagnosis. Employers, unions, lawyers and government departments, together with employee groups, self-help groups and health professionals, all circulated these pamphlets which focused on the early diagnosis and prevention of RSI.

DISTURBANCES OF FUNCTION LEADING TO DISABILITY IN SOMATIZATION

Abnormalities of function as well as sensation are essential for the diagnosis of somatization.

All personal needs can still be attended to with the affected limb while, at the same time, the person is unable to perform a specific task. A cramp subject could play the piano but could not type, might knit and sew but be unable to press a typewriter key (old-fashioned or electronic) without experiencing pain or palsy.

While purporting to demonstrate that a hand or finger cannot be moved or an object cannot be held, cramp subjects use the same flexor and extensor muscles quite normally to maintain posture. The level of disability is more severe than in the organically impaired. The cramp subject cannot cook and clean without feeling it, whereas a person with a broken arm uses the healthy one.

Clinical signs in somatization can be turned on at will. Jerks and spasms can be imitated. Where spasm has been measured in hysteria subjects it is produced at 12 cycles per second and this frequency is easily reproduced by the voluntary clenching of flexors and extensors together (McEvedy & Beard 1970).

DISABILITIES

The jargon-ridden paradigm-based presentation of symptoms is a clue to somatization. Cramp subjects recite the disabilities that have been suggested to them. Familiar with the RSI prevention guides, they become educated by repeated examinations and support groups where they exchange symptoms and histories. The list of selectively reported disabilities that was promoted (such as holding a telephone in the course of non-typing duties, using hair-rollers, or dropping objects) has sometimes identified a subject's specific source of RSI information. Symptoms that have attracted the sympathetic attention of an expert in RSI are emphasised to the next medical examiner, together with learnt attribution theories.

RESPONSE OF CRAMP SUBJECTS TO TREATMENT

Cramp subjects seemed willing to undergo any prescribed pharmacological, medical, surgical, physical or alternative therapies. They praised the doctors who had treated them with so little success. 'It helped at the time but the symptoms came back [hours, days, weeks] later' evidenced a placebo response. They admitted to knowing that the same treatment had been ineffective in their friends.

Treatment failure was reported for acupuncture, cervical traction and cortisone, exercises, electrical stimulation, hot wax baths, iodine, copper, local hydro-cortisone, rest, non-steroidal anti-inflammatory drugs, manipulation, physiotherapy, plaster, slings, splints, supports, surgery, ultrasonic therapy and vitamin B-12. Some potent centrally acting analgesics gave temporary relief, but no more than was to be expected of mood-elevating drugs — they did not provide a cure.

Functional symptoms did not respond to immobilisation; rather, their response tended to be paradoxical. Many subjects reported that their symptoms got worse after they had been prescribed a week's rest at home. Symptoms crossed into a formerly unaffected arm during the first weeks of the disability, after a claimant had been sent home to rest, just as had been published in guidebooks. Claimants volunteered that crossover of symptoms had been caused by compensatory overuse of the non-affected arm to protect the affected one. Sardonic comments were made to the effect that if overuse symptoms occurred from normal domestic activity they would have been common knowledge and would not have had to wait to be discovered in the Australian workforce in the 1980s.

Although cramp subjects' responses to rest and to physical therapies are unpredictable or paradoxical, some doctors were easily deceived by spontaneous remissions in all disorders. As Hendrick Wulff (1976) explained, this illusion allowed doctors to persist in their administration of physical remedies even when they were no longer useful.

The amount or type of work done before development of symptoms was not constant, varying between years and days, and how long the person was affected ranged from moments to years.

Disregard for circumstantial evidence, including the situation in which the symptom arose, left a clinical phenomenon for which an organic mechanism could not be postulated.

8

SYMPTOMS, REMEDIES AND PREDICAMENTS

*What we observe is not nature itself, but nature
exposed to our method of questioning.*

Werner Heisenberg, *Physics and Philosophy*

At the request of third parties in five states, I interviewed 319 litigating subjects with arm symptoms in the period between October 1984 and April 1991. In all 319 cases, I recorded the mode of onset, the medical interpretations offered, the treatments applied and the beliefs and attribution theories of cramp subjects, in counterpoint with their concurrent social histories and predicaments. In April 1991, these 319 files were listed in alphabetical order and 100 were selected by random number screen to create a group of 100, which is referred to as G100. The case histories of the first 20 of them, which I have called G20, are documented in Chapter 11.

This survey is qualitative rather than quantitative in its thrust. The diagnoses of somatization or functional disorder were made when symptoms did not submit to a disease diagnosis, when they accorded with the subjects' belief system about them and when they were preceded by obvious stress, a need for respite or a conflict of obligations. Somatization occurred on its own or, in about 20 per cent of my sample, it complicated other organic arm problems, most of which were not related to the occupation.

The claimants were predominantly women (97 per cent) and aged 19–59 years. No age group was over-represented, but fewer claimants were older than 45. This reflected the ages of women in the workforce.

The claimants were experiencing high levels of demand from competing responsibilities. Their lives revealed predicaments that demanded attention to needs and responsibilities. They laboured under extraordinary levels of personal stress, compared with a census population. One-third of them had significant health problems.

The survey uncovered the practices of a number medically qualified, high status practitioners who had adopted the injury theory of RSI in its entirely, just as it was taught by government-appointed people and organisations. These doctors genuinely believed in what they were doing, as they were responding to the orthodoxy of the time.

The information collected concerns a relatively brief period in the history of Australian medical practice when it came under the influence of a social movement. This survey is unusual in that it is unrepeatable. There might never again be a possibility of setting up a study to examine the clinical transactions between cramp subjects and their physicians. Had they known that their diagnosis and treatment behaviour patterns were being observed, doctors might have changed both. Prospective studies would cause them to do just that.

There is no literature on epidemic somatization in a situation where compensation is being paid for it. There is, as yet, no category of epidemic somatization in *Index Medicus*. The findings and commentary here might not hold true for a sample of litigating cramp subjects outside the period of the 1980s and 1990s. Beliefs and attendant clinical practices, which had been around for 150 years, are probably still being offered to cramp subjects around the world.

Long after RSI had gone away in other jurisdictions, new cases of it emerged in the Commonwealth public service sector, which was covered by its own legislation, Comcare.

No comment can be made about the practices of the broader community of medical practitioners.

VALIDITY ISSUES

My survey was not a life-event study and it makes no claim to that cumbersome category of inquiry. The point of reference was the presentation of a specific somatoform disorder, an occupation neurosis.

Claimant data were compared with person data available from the census. This disclosed some very large differences in the incidence of certain life events. Patient data, commonly used as a control in studies of somatization and other mental disorders, would be different again. The conclusion is that RSI is more likely to be related to life events, stresses and conflicts than to any identified aspects of tasks or occupations.

Acts of malingering, lying, withholding strategic information and faking weakness were apparent in at least 20 per cent of subjects. Some claimants could have been making symptoms up entirely, embellishing or falsely reporting old and familiar symptoms from an earlier period of affliction. Some may have been reporting more symptoms than they had experienced or some that they had just read about.

Some deceived by failing to report events that provided cogent reasons for stopping work: the birth of children, overseas travel to see sick parents and other crises. One woman, with whom I had two interviews, avoided telling me that she developed RSI at the same time as she had adopted a child from abroad, but she had taken the child to another doctor who made a note of the five-year-old in the waiting room. The existence of serious health problems was frequently denied and other work and study activities were not revealed. Sometimes information emerged by chance or through secondary sources or when a fully investigated case went to court. Some subjects claimed, while being examined, that they could not handle an object that weighed less than the handbags they had carried in to their appointments.

Malingering behaviours presented themselves in subjects who, at the time that they went off work, had good reasons for somatizing. This might have been months or years before the interview. They had not gone back to work and seemed to be trapped in the sick role. Some had no jobs to go back to and they were studying, caring for children or helping in family businesses. Some claimants avoided examination altogether by taking the position that private matters such as health status, family and marital difficulties, sexual liaisons, alcohol use were none of the medical examiner's concern, as the injury was in the arms.

The opportunities to malinger were inexhaustible. I chose to ignore them in favour of testing the hypothesis that the claimant had not suffered an injury but was experiencing a disorder caused by her beliefs and desires. In a strict causation model, or in any litigation that demanded any standard at all, hysteria and malingering are not compensable as injuries as neither can possibly be caused by a physical event. Being given a diagnosis of physical injury, where none exists, provides an opportunity for action. Opportunities are not causes.

THE REMUNERATION OF DOCTORS

In Australia, medical treatment is available for a minimal cost on Medicare, the national health system. This provides for subsidised fees in a doctor's office, and public hospitals offer free hospitalisation. Psychologists, counsellors, physiotherapists, occupational therapists, osteopaths and chiropractors all charge fees that do not attract a subsidy. Most have a significant income stream from treating injured claimants who attract third-party payments. Public hospitals are staffed by staff specialists and visiting consultants. About 20–30 per cent of the population is insured for private hospitalisation, but the uninsured cannot pay fees for surgical services that require operating theatres. Staff specialists, junior doctors or consultants provide services for them.

In the United Kingdom, subjects received surgical and physiotherapeutic interventions in hospitals run by the National Health Service. Staff surgeons had nothing personal to gain except a small fee for writing a report. The desire for a fee was not a motivating factor; rather, physicians and surgeons did what they did with RSI subjects because that was what they were trained to do. They are expected to see problems through a medical gaze.

WHO DIAGNOSED AND TREATED RSI PATIENTS?

This study could not be set up prospectively, as it would be impossible to know where the diagnosis would be made. The claimants did not attend their regular general practitioners so family doctors rarely diagnosed RSI. One woman had accompanied her sick mother to an appointment, and was given a certificate for RSI by her mother's doctor. The mother was no longer able to care for the grandchild. Another woman took her sick child to the doctor, casually mentioned a sore wrist and was given a certificate for herself. Having a certificate for RSI freed each woman to care for her child. In four of G20, the claimant told me that the doctor had become involved on behalf of arm symptoms that were not the reason she had consulted him, and that she had left with a diagnosis of a gynaecological problem and a certificate for workers' compensation. The incidental diagnosis of RSI allowed the patient to take time off on full pay without using her sick leave.

Many claimants had actively sought out the sick role. In one study, 20 of 60 RSI subjects changed their doctor at least once, and some up to four times, during their 'pilgrimage of pain' before they found one who 'knew about RSI' (Reid et al. 1991).

Table 8.1 Time off work

Time off at time of interview	Number of subjects	Number back to work
0–2 months	14	10
3–6 months inclusive	11	4
7–12 months	19	3
13–24 months	23	
25–36 months	14	1
37–48 months	9	
49–60 months	5	
60 months or more	5	
Total	100	18

The early years of the epidemic were characterised by long periods of work disability. Table 8.1 indicates that at the time of interview, 86 of G100 had three months or more off work on compensation, 75 more than six months, 55 had more than a year, and five had five years or more. Only 18 were back at work when I saw them.

DIAGNOSTIC PROCEDURES

Blood tests were commonly done but rarely reported in the files. Thermography went through a brief vogue and yielded results that were rapidly consigned to the category of artefact (Awerbuch 1991a, 1991b).

X-rays and bone scans were given almost as a routine and, as symptoms moved from place to place and from one arm to the other, more of them were ordered. Bone scans of wrist bones and epicondyles showed an increase or decrease in bone density, seemingly at random. Scans yielded artefacts that failed to account for symptoms. Needle biopsies of forearm muscles were commonly performed, but no results were reported.

Nerve conduction studies on the median and ulnar nerves were routinely carried out in many centres and slow nerves were used as a justification for performing surgery.

CLAIMANT DATA

Of G100, 16 were typists, stenographers and data-processing operators, while 22 did occasional or light keyboard work and included telephonists. Four used a pen to write but did no keyboard work, seven did clerical work and answered phones but did not use keyboards. They were receptionists who took messages and two were managers. Process workers numbered 25 and a further 24 were builders, cleaners, a caretaker, a librarian some police and some teachers.

Table 8.2 lists health problems of G100 concurrent with RSI.

Table 8.2 Health problems concurrent with RSI

Patient age	Concurrent problems
20	Multiple recurrent inexplicable illnesses: somatization disorder
21	Injured neck in a motor vehicle accident months before leaving with RSI
24	Ear and eye troubles (unspecified but troublesome kind)
24	Anorexia nervosa
24	Miscarriage, bunions surgery anaemia, hysterectomy (all while receiving compensation for RSI)*
25	Surgery to enable pregnancy*
25	2 laparoscopies, conceived and bore a child (all while receiving compensation for RSI)*
28	Recurrent bouts of undiagnosed abdominal pain and major depression
31	Chronic cholecystitis, pregnant, wearing a collar (recent motor vehicle accident)
31	Schizophrenia
32	Litigating separately for a fall at work
32	Grossly overweight, hiatus hernia, barbiturate and codeine addiction
33	Motor vehicle accident
34	Myxoedema and hypertension
36	Severe depressive illness
36	Abusing alcohol and attempted suicide
38	Problems from old neck injury
38	Motor vehicle accident after leaving work
40	Hysterectomy and oophorectomy; on return, she developed RSI and left

40	Prostate problems and proctalgia fugax
40	Simultaneous litigation (traffic accident after she left work with RSI)
41	Gynaecological problems resulting in anaemia needing surgery*
41	Gynaecological problems resulting in anaemia
41	Influenza, viral infection re-formulated as 'RSI'
43	Suffering from the effects of a fall at work
43	Positive rheumatoid factor, rheumatoid arthritis, depression Bells palsy
45	Gynaecological problems, anaemia necessitating an hysterectomy*
45	Symptomatic mitral valve disease
48	Gynaecological problems resulting in anaemia and hysterectomy*
51	Arthritis in the neck
52	Generalised osteoarthritis with Heberden's nodes
52	Needed and had surgery for urinary incontinence*
59	Had an aortic graft for an aortic aneurism on compensation*

* These patients went on to have operations for other reasons while receiving compensation for RSI.

Health impairment was a well-documented precipitant for cramp. Thirty-three subjects revealed health problems and eight had undergone surgery for problems unrelated to arm symptoms within weeks of going off on workers' compensation. Normally, they would have taken sick leave.

Six had readily diagnosable psychiatric disorders of a major kind. The organic status of neck problems was rarely substantiated. Neck pain had its origins in old car accidents, but it was not unusual for a claimant to indulge in double dipping by attributing neck and arm pain to the car accident and, after settlement, to RSI.

Claimants under-reported prior health problems. I expected to find a concentration of somatoform disorders, but this did not emerge. However, when I examined 20 RSI claimants in England, they also routinely denied prior medical histories. In the United Kingdom, however, it was normal practice to obtain records of litigating subjects and full records were available because of National Health Service arrangements. I found that virtually all RSI claimants in the United Kingdom had minimised their health history at interview or had avoided giving any account of it at all. Most had deceived me and other examiners on the subject of earlier symptomatic states attracting unproductive investigations. Nearly all of them could have been diagnosed as recurrent somatizers. The co-existence of somatoform disorder in the Australian sample would be expected to be very high, but histories were not disclosed.

More than 20 of the Australian G100 sample were concurrently, or had been previously, involved in litigation concerning a health issue, a motor vehicle accident claim, a period of disability, or were in pursuit of early superannuation on medical grounds or had previously claimed workers' compensation payments for more than six months. This was a large proportion.

PRESENTATION OF CASES

Onset of symptoms was different in every case and it seemed to be at random, with pain, palsy, paralysis, paraesthesiae or sensations in the back, neck, shoulder, arm or forearm, on the dorsal or ventral aspect or on the medial or lateral aspect of the arm, difficulties in manipulation, pain, loss of sensation or cramp. Some people experienced escalating discomfort, others had sudden onset at work, at home, at night, while hanging out washing or at the breakfast table. One woman came into work after a harrowing row at home about her husband's gambling and found her word-processing hand to be palsied. The industrial magistrate rejected my evidence and gave her compensation.

In general, subjects gave their history in the language of the guides, attributed it to doctors' advice and recited their symptoms and disabilities as if from a crib. In such cases, the symptoms and their causes were offered, as it were, in one breath, in a pre-wrapped package.

Few claimants were interested in alternative views or explanations and most met any new information with bland disdain. They made it clear that they wanted the remedies that had been negotiated for them, which at that time included long periods of compensable leave. The predominant emotional tone was one of entitlement. This was combined with an expectation that the medical examiner would not easily sanction their demands.

In the textbook case, the somatizing patient displays an overabundance of feelings of entitlement, as well as compulsive, paranoid or passive aggressive traits. These characteristics were evident in the G100 sample. Entitlement was encouraged by pamphlets, guides to prevention, union delegates, ministers of state, feminists, legal advisers, counsellors and the subjects' preferred doctors, as well as by the context in which the examinations took place.

Some claimants argued their entitlement so strongly they created a passable imitation of paranoid certainty. In general, those with the strongest feelings of entitlement and the highest level of political motivation displayed fewer and less cogent personal reasons to develop and maintain symptoms. These women were the intellectuals, the carriers of the ideologies of 'RSI as a social movement' (Arksey 1994) and they proudly recited their unions' goals to change their working conditions.

THE CLAIMANTS' PREDICAMENTS

Predicaments have been defined as painful social situations or circumstances, complex, unstable, morally charged and varying in their import in time and place. They are readily discernible from a good history and they are rich in conflicts (Taylor 1985). A predicament encompasses not only the stress, conflict or life event operating at the time, but also the opportunities that the subject has available to her for coping with it as well as constraints. Predicaments are understood intuitively and empathically or they are not understood at all.

Personal problems and disruptive life events were common to all and, more often than not, had come in quick succession. Distress seemed to be cumulative. Definable life events such as marriage, pregnancy, marital break-up, bereavement, personal and family illnesses contained in these predicaments could be counted, and some of these could be compared with the five-yearly Commonwealth census data. Other stresses also occurred more often in the G100 sample than one would expect, involving events that occur twice in an individual's life (such as death of parents) and some that do not even occur in everyone's life (such as building a house).

Life events were categorised as personal health impairment, the formation of new relationships, pregnancy, responding to the needs of children, relationship difficulties, serious illness in a family member, occupational problem, being engaged in other activities, and a predicament in which working was no longer financially rewarding.

Three claimants were experiencing five categories of event each, 3 were experiencing four, 21 were experiencing three, 30 were experiencing two and 36 were experiencing only one event. This covered 93 subjects. Two more claimants were experiencing personal difficulties that were not so easily coded. No reasons for adopting illness behaviour were uncovered in two subjects, and three had easily identified physical conditions in their arms and no functional overlay.

Personal health impairment was the most common, accounting for 33 cases. Women went off work for hysterectomies, miscarriages and for surgery to enable pregnancy. Next most common were traumatic disorders consequent on motor accidents and falls. These were followed by psychological problems, depression, psychosis, anorexia nervosa, addiction and a previously recognised tendency towards recurrent somatization, then various arthritic and metabolic illnesses or serious cardiovascular disorders. Nine subjects entered hospital for surgery for unrelated health problems within weeks of going off work with RSI. They would have been aware of their intentions before they presented certificates for workers' compensation.

Thirteen subjects were in the process of forming new relationships that involved a change of domicile. Seven got married within weeks of going off with RSI, three more became engaged while in receipt of compensation payments and two had married and moved house not long before making their claims. One had formed a relationship in another town, too far away to commute, and had moved there just before claiming compensation.

Seven marriages in 100 people represents a higher rate than the 1986 and 1991 census rates for marriage that are recorded in the relevant age groups. In the census figures, the rate of marriage is given by decile and it ranges between one and two per cent. Cramp subjects were much more likely to be getting married than was the census population. The rate of formation of de facto relationships was not recorded in the census.

Eleven subjects went off work pregnant and more went off, never to return, within days or weeks of coming back after maternity leave. Most reported that they had experienced symptoms before they left to have their babies. The census rate of pregnancy is 3.97 per cent. Some people failed to reveal pregnancies when they were seen for the first time, and these were discovered later. I suspect that there were more than 11, as I found out about most of these after the interview and as I had so many anecdotal reports to the effect that everyone knew someone who went off with RSI and was pregnant.

Seventeen women were responding to the demands of their children. The pregnancy was not the only stress that precipitated the symptoms, but having other children at home made it more difficult to go back to work. Other women had lost childminders, grandparents, neighbours or friends and had no choice but to stay home.

The sample contained 72 married people and six in de facto relationships. Eleven of the marriages were in the process of breaking up when the subject left work and had already broken up by the time of my interview. The annual rate of divorce in the general population is 1.26 per cent of marriages per year. Permanent separation before divorce occurred in close conjunction with the development of RSI many times more often than in the census population.

Two of the married subjects had separated and had reconciled. A further four claimants reported being desperately unhappy in their marriages. Three of the six de facto couples were in the process of breaking up. Other relationship problems also involved separation from significant others: a son, a lover, a fiancé.

Twenty-one people were coded as having an occupational problem. This number included those who were facing retrenchment because their workplace was closing. Some disliked their supervisors or their jobs or were discontented because they saw their tasks as menial and inappropriate. Some were over-educated and bored. One, but likely more, had formed an injudicious sexual liaison at work. I excluded from the occupational problem category the recited complaints concerning the dangers of keyboard work, the faults of furniture, doing too much and not having enough to do. Occupational tasks were common to all and had not affected their neighbours. I did include overwork causing endless unwanted overtime.

Six subjects were enrolled in tertiary studies, part-time. At that time, six per cent of the Australian population was enrolled in tertiary institutions, with full-time students comprising half that number. Part-time students were over-represented, possibly by a factor of two. Some had been studying part-time and became full-time students when they won compensation payments. Having entered university on a disabled quota, they continued to receive rehabilitation allowances. One was studying the violin although she claimed inability to type.

Five women were engaged in supervising the building or renovation of their houses.

Twelve women had found it uneconomic or senseless to work. Some had just redeemed settlements from motor vehicle accident claims and they stopped work on compensation certificates for RSI very soon after. The husbands of five women had become eligible for a social security pension that would have been reduced on a dollar-for-dollar basis if their wives continued to receive an income. Others stopped work, taking compensation, after they made their last mortgage payment or after the last child left home.

If compensation had not been available simply for the report of symptoms, many of these women might have made other arrangements to have children, spouses and parents cared for, or they would have left work to pursue their obligations and other interests.

Although part-time work for those who want it might provide a solution to such problems, the finding in Telecom Australia was that part-time employees were more likely than full-time workers to develop RSI.

Taking another look at these findings, it seemed that 70 per cent of the claimants were dealing with losses and, in some cases, were grieving them. The most common loss was that of health (33) and some of this was transient. This was followed by the actual or impending loss of a relationship with a significant other, either through separation or that person's dementia or death (26). The threat of losing a job was significant (10). In those cases where the husband had been injured or had become ill, the loss of his working and hence economic capacity affected eight subjects. Other losses were more abstract but quite common: the loss of religious faith, of hope and opportunities and of idealised beliefs about people close to them.

Sixty per cent of the sample could not possibly have continued to work at the same time as attending to their considerable responsibilities and obligations to family members. Women were responsible for children or sick relatives and finding others to care for them was neither possible nor affordable.

A new kind of leave is called for, a kind suited to helping women weather family crises without losing their jobs.

9

PERCEPTIONS AND RESPONSES

Neurosis has an absolute genius for malingering.
There is no illness which it cannot counterfeit perfectly.
If it is capable of deceiving the doctor,
how should it fail to deceive the patient?

Marcel Proust (1921)

Various interesting, idiosyncratic and self-serving beliefs underpinned the activities of medical and paramedical professionals, unions, sociologists and philosophers, claimants and the media in the Australian RSI epidemic.

The affirmative side of the debate, that RSI is an injury, was argued from the clinics and the academies by strategically placed medical administrators, leading professors, medical educators and occupational health specialists. There were also the moral entrepreneurs, clinicians who influenced politicians, trade unions, the courts and institutions and, all together, they caused many thousands of people to enter the sick role and to litigate.

Interest in the RSI controversy was not limited to medical and paramedical professionals and psychologists who had expertise in the diagnostic assessment of cramp subjects. Debate about the epidemic also continued in journals of sociology and health studies and in the popular press.

A new bureaucracy of RSI experts emerged: RSI co-ordinating officers, nurses, physiotherapists and occupational therapists. Schoolchildren were informed of the official and dominant view of its physical origins. Teachers in secretarial colleges rapped slouching students on the knuckles, telling them that they would get RSI from their bad posture. Trade unions and lawyers advertised their services in winning compensation.

Physicians promoted their particular models of explanation within different theoretical frameworks and their clinical activities were based on their beliefs.

THE VIEWS OF MEDICAL PROFESSIONALS

The most influential proponents of RSI were the authors of the original papers: Ferguson, Stone, Browne, Nolan and Faithfull. They were joined by others operating from various workers' and occupational health clinics. Those whose practices centred on RSI referred their patients to like-minded professionals. It would have caused mutual embarrassment to do otherwise.

The earliest medical theories postulated the use, overuse or failure to use certain muscles (Browne et al. 1984). Attribution theories expanded as new ones were devised on a case-by-case basis.

Pockets of distinctive formulations and treatments were found in each of the states of Australia. These were often published, as breakthroughs in refereed journals, or as letters to the editor, and they were immediately taken up in RSI newsletters and the lay press. All added to the increasingly confused body of medical opinion. Such information was immediately promoted as further evidence of knowledge of a physical origin for the symptoms, whereas it was nothing of the sort. This demonstrated the power of medical pronouncements.

Some formulations were only medical in the sense that they used words like 'inflammation', 'something-itis' or 'injury', thus suggesting the syndrome was accessible to medical cure. The diversity of criticisms, commentaries and interventions suggested that there were as many organic theories of RSI as there were theorists. This fulfilled the expectation of Illich (1974, 1975), who had characterised medicine as 'an expansionist profession that turns ills into illnesses, to be treated by doctors until persons lose their ability to cope with indisposition or even with discomfort'.

Some physicians who became involved in treating RSI believed that there were different lesions in each case. They then took the position that it was appropriate to treat symptoms of RSI by methods that had been successful in other cases where the symptoms had been similar. In effect, they treated the functional mimic as if it were the real disease that it suggested. Multiple and non-specific lesions were diagnosed.

Non-steroidal anti-inflammatory drugs were widely prescribed. These drugs can cause internal bleeding and in 1992 it was estimated that 200 fatalities a year could be attributed to their use (Cooke 1992). Modern anti-inflammatory medication is not so dangerous to the stomach.

Very little of the discourse concerned the hypothetical lesion in RSI, except in so far as there was general agreement that there was no consistent pathology.

Medical experts divided into those who saw RSI as a condition of task-related traumatic origin and those who had other theories about how it came into existence. The epidemic somatization, mass hysteria, theory was only one of these. Family doctors and psychiatrists were aware that stress made some people sick. Many physicians attempted sociological and political explanations of the epidemic, describing conditions that might lead to epidemic somatization or illness behaviour.

Only a small proportion of medical practitioners became involved in what they believed to be the prevention and treatment of RSI. However, as the statistics revealed, they maintained their patients in the sick role for long periods.

Doctors who were prepared to diagnose within an injury paradigm rapidly made themselves known. They clustered in groups, adopted certain beliefs about the physical causes of RSI and acted as magnets for somatizing patients by providing certificates and explanations as well as remedies.

OCCUPATIONAL HEALTH CLINICS

Industrial health clinics were set up in industrial areas and competed for the clientele of suburban GPs. Such blatant politicisation as their practice names implied was new in Australia.

Workers were referred by shop stewards and union delegates and, in some cases, at the height of the reporting period in 1984, these third parties made appointments. Entrepreneurial doctors gave public lectures inviting potential claimants, and some published articles in paramedical journals which publicised their support for popular attribution theories and suggested the promise of salvation from the dangers of work. Representatives of clinics lectured in the workplace and distributed pamphlets on early detection.

The Trade Union Medical Centre in Sydney reported that more than 800 RSI patients had come through its doors in 1984–85

(Drury 1985). At least two state-funded teaching hospitals (Sydney Hospital and Westmead) opened occupational health clinics and administered physical remedies to subjects complaining of RSI.

RHEUMATOLOGISTS

Rheumatologists led the debate both for and against RSI as an injury. Their interpretations rarely fell within their own body of knowledge and they had no cures to offer, but this did not deter them from what Freidson had called 'tinkering'.

A leading critic of the injury concept was Dr Peter Brooks, at that time a professor of rheumatology. He commented on the inevitability of muscular fatigue and discomfort in the course of work (Brooks 1986a, 1986b, 1988) and proposed that the less presumptive diagnosis of 'regional pain syndrome' be adopted. He agreed with Cleland (1987) that the condition was a model of social iatrogenesis.

Bowing to this influence, the Royal Australian College of Physicians published a memorandum to the effect that the name RSI should be changed (RACP 1986).

Mark Awerbuch, the Adelaide rheumatologist who claimed that he had coined the term kangaroo paw, developed a model of sensory dysfunction, a theory compatible with that of somatization (Awerbuch 1987).

In England, Dr Richard Pearson provided expert evidence in the case of *Mughal v Reuters* (1993). He described his academic connections as 'The Musicians and Keyboard Clinic' and the 'Rheumatology Department of St Bartholemew's Hospital'. He wrote many reports on British RSI claimants. He exposed all his patients to his beliefs. He provided them with lists of the disabilities that they could expect with RSI and information concerning activities they could and could not perform and how they might be assisted by various gadgets. Judge Prosser pointed out that Pearson was a trained pharmacologist and a self-styled rheumatologist and criticised him for orchestrating a large amount of treatment for the journalist, Rafiq Mughal.

Pearson wrote about 'intellectually sound principles' of management. Pearson ascribed his failure to treat the condition successfully to what he called 'barriers to the management of repetition injuries'. He wrote that RSI was poorly described in standard textbooks, that it interfaced between many specialities, including neurology, orthopaedics and rheumatology, that these were unhappy patients who needed special handling, that doctors feared involvement in the provision of medicolegal reports, that few physiotherapists, other than those whom he had trained, were able to provide treatment and, finally, that RSI ran a prolonged course and its management was time consuming, needing much liaison.

Dr Richard Wigley made several unrelated criticisms that were published in *The Neurogenic Hypothesis* (Quintner & Elvey 1991). He said that the authors had omitted to mention that weakness preceded the pain syndrome. He warned against extrapolating from patients seen at tertiary referral clinics to those in the working community. He pointed out that nervous tension increased muscle tension and fed back to produce a self-perpetuating pain cycle; relaxation could break this cycle. He referred to a study in which three groups of patients were mixed together: normal controls and those diagnosed as suffering from myofascial pain syndrome and those who had been diagnosed as having fibromyalgia. Musculoskeletal specialists who were asked to diagnose them blind made an attempt that produced humbling results.

Dr John Quintner, a rheumatologist in Western Australia, took a view in favour of occupational causation. Although he did not uphold its rheumatological basis, his position at the beginning of the epidemic was that RSI was the result of undefined problems in the region of the brachial plexus caused by poor posture (Quintner et al. 1986). In conjunction with R. L. Elvey, a physiotherapist, he devised and reported on the Brachial Plexus Stretch Test, by means of which they claimed to be able to diagnose damage to nervous tissue that had been stretched by the patient's occupational activities (Elvey 1988). The validity of this test was much contested, but Dr Quintner took the position that it was 'part of the orthopaedic examination'.

The brachial plexus is located at the top of the armpit, where spinal nerves from the cervical and high thoracic regions come together and then emerge as the nerves that supply the arm. These nerves are a combination of various spinal roots, and a good knowledge of neuroanatomy is required to repair them in the event of a tear. The combination of spinal roots, which emerge as each nerve, is known, so there is no reason to suppose that vague symptoms are somehow related to the brachial plexus. Indeed, hand surgeons and neurologists would pride themselves on their ability to identify the exact position of a tear or a tumour by the clinical signs that such a lesion would cause at some distance from it.

Quintner, however, could not concede that specific entrapment syndromes resulted in specific neurological deficits. In this regard he joined a group of surgeons who operated unsuccessfully on many patients' wrists for entrapment syndromes, although Quintner did not do surgery.

Quintner and Elvey went on to publish a monograph, *The Neurogenic Hypothesis of RSI, together with 'Commentaries'* (Quintner & Elvey 1991). At that time, their hypothesis involved the conjecture that peripheral nerves had been stretched or trapped at various sites along their courses and thereby injured by repetitive work.

Dr Quintner invoked the Japanese name from the 1970s, occupational cervico-brachial disorder. Although less presumptive than RSI, the term still incorporated the notion that the context in which the symptoms had developed, work, was also their cause. Dr Quintner made no claims to providing successful therapies; rather, he saw neuropathic pains as notoriously unresponsive to treatment and the patients as currently incurable, meriting his empathy and support.

Later Quintner went on to criticise me and others whom he called 'psychalgic fundamentalists' who, he believed, made the fundamental error of refusing to accept that the widespread pain and other sensory phenomena, such as tingling and numbness, that characterised RSI could ever be explained in terms of bodily dysfunction (Quintner 2000). He saw it as a monumental leap into the mind of the patient to attempt to provide an explanation in terms of contemporary psychiatric diagnoses.

Quintner thought somatization to be a 'wonderful label as it could embrace every poorly understood clinical problem, as did fibromyalgia'. He did not differentiate somatization from imaginary pain and implied that these diagnoses involved a demoralising interpretation, to wit, 'It's all in your mind, dear!'

Quintner wrote to me in 2000, citing a number of research studies which he said had 'filled the knowledge gap that you (and we) encountered in 1985/6', and offered a third explanatory model, in which clinical phenomena originated in the nervous system. He cited a number of text book descriptions of this phenomenon.

Quintner insisted that my explanatory model had not been useful to him and others who had closely examined the problem of diffuse upper limb pain from a neurobiological standpoint. By his account, the debate had moved on but my views had stayed put. Furthermore, my views had remained untestable and therefore irrefutable. He believed that the opposing views were such that they were not able to be reconciled.

This view of undiagnosable symptoms as being somehow mediated through the peripheral nervous system was consistent with that of Cullen (1710–90) and his original eighteenth century notion of neuroses. This predated the connection that was later made between such undiagnosable symptoms and the emotional states that accompanied them.

Quintner remained an injury theorist, one who conceptualised that peripheral tissues, most probably nerves, had somehow been affected by occupational use.

In late 1992, a Sydney group of active believers in a theory of traumatic origin for RSI constructed a new theory of pain production (Cohen et al. 1992). This theory was based on 'central sensitisation of nociceptive function', on which they further published (1992, 1993), and they sought to explain the clinical phenomena to which the label RSI had been attached. In their model, poor posture, movements that had been performed or static loading were believed to have had a role in the sensitisation of tissues. Movements and muscle actions were assumed to have caused some peripheral but unidentified physiological change.

They found the injury theory of RSI to be unsatisfactory, but found the psychogenic interpretation to be tautological. Cohen maintained that control subjects were required only to test a theory, not to propose one. Furthermore, he considered it to be not ethically or practically possible to use, as controls, workers from the same industry who have not yet developed pain.

This group denied that hysteria or somatization theories were valid and saw psychiatrists as dismissing their patients' pain with terms they interpreted as pejorative. Cohen also wrote in 2000 to tell me that it was a pity that my research had stopped in 1992, as neuroscience had progressed since that time. He suspected my book would be out of date and of little interest. He asked 'By contrast, how can you test theories of psychogenic pathogenesis?'

My correspondence with Quintner and Cohen reactivated an ongoing and sometimes acrimonious debate between two groups of experts who made different assumptions about not only RSI, but many other syndromes for which no bodily causes could be found. Psychiatrists know these as the functional somatic syndromes (Barsky 1999) and they include multiple chemical sensitivity, the sick building syndrome, the side-effects of silicone breast implants, the Gulf War syndrome, chronic whiplash, myalgic encephalomyelitis, chronic fatigue syndrome, dental galvanism and fibromyalgia. This debate polarised the two groups of experts aligned with their paradigmatic assumptions.

My position is that these rival groups of experts address quite different aspects of RSI. The somatic theorists advance that something happens in the arms of afflicted workers to sensitise tissues to pain. They concern themselves with a theory of peripheral origin and peripheral pathology, one that has not yet been identified. Quintner initially speculated about nerves, in what he called the neurogenic hypothesis of pain production, and Cohen hypothesised about what might be going on in muscles or tissues.

Somatic theorists assume that the body has to have something wrong with it for it to send signals that the mind registers as informing of local problems. Their deliberations concern possible mechanisms of pain production in the tissues of the arm, presumptively caused by occupational tasks.

But peripheral theories concerning mechanisms of pain production accommodate neither the epidemiology of RSI nor the epidemic of claims for it. Nor do they accommodate its changing and mobile symptomatology, nor the coexistence of emotional difficulties nor the effects of massive stressors and life events. No evidence has ever been presented that those who had RSI had done anything differently from those who did not have it. Indeed statistics from Telecom Australia resemble those from the epidemic of telegraphists' cramp in the early twentieth century. All deny any connection with quantity of work done. The converse is true: there is an inverse relationship between the amount of work done and the likelihood of claiming for RSI. Nor was pain a constant complaint; rather, patients complained of a variety of sensations, pins and needles and numbness, hot and cold, and symptoms went on beyond the natural history of the lesions they complicated or mimicked. In almost every case, transient and variable weakness, sometimes to the point of palsy or paralysis, accompanied disorder of sensation in a way that could not be explained by anatomy or biology.

The search for the physical basis of hysteria has been going on for 300 years. Treatable organic causes now appear improbable.

Somatization theory is a theory of causation by mental events. It explains how the body is experienced when certain psychosocial conditions prevail. Somatization might accommodate those clinical situations where a nerve or even a spinal cord has been cut or where a person has continued having feelings in a limb from which the nerves have been severed. Somatization might also account for instances of phantom limb pain, which is pain experienced in a limb that has been amputated.

Somatization theory looks at how symptoms are influenced and delineated by what a patient believes or fears is wrong. It explains how popular beliefs affect a body part that the patient believes to be diseased, whether it is or is not. Somatization is a central phenomenon, mediated by the mind and those entities that impinge on the mind, ideas and beliefs, needs and desires. Pain is conceptualised as referred onto the affected part: general hypersensitivity follows and random clinical signs are to be found, most commonly those of disuse. Epidemics of symptoms follow the circulation of ideas, as in education and prevention campaigns, and symptoms afflict the anxious and depressed.

People who have been physically injured battle to overcome their disabilities. Those with RSI complacently accepted and displayed, as the inevitable consequence of their condition, a level of disability that would have been catastrophic had it come from a stroke or the like.

Somatization theory does not concern what might be happening in the body parts where the symptoms are experienced, what is happening in the chest wall or heart muscle when a person has stress-related chest pain, nor what is happening in the knees when they feel weak in response to a fright. Similarly, when there is glove and stocking or body quadrant distribution of pain, somatization theory does not tell a researcher what tissues should be examined nor by what test.

The vulnerable emerged and felt entitled to adopt the new, socially constructed illness because it provided resolution, albeit temporarily, for their predicaments. The presentation of cramp subjects is completely different from that of the organically impaired.

PSYCHIATRISTS

In 1986 I published the earliest substantial challenge to the RSI model in the *Medical Journal of Australia* (Lucire 1986). This paper, 'Neurosis in the workplace', was held up more than a year by referees (specialists in occupational health), who labelled its contents 'idiosyncratic', notwithstanding their being consistent with the *International Classification of Disease*. I requested referees in psychiatry and the paper was published. It identified an epidemic of somatization in the form of writers' cramp and I pursued an investigation into how iatrogenesis on a grand scale had occurred.

Dr David Bell, a psychiatrist and experienced medical examiner, criticised the construction and notion of RSI and concluded that it was an example of clinical and social iatrogenesis, an iatrogenic epidemic of simulated injury together with fabrication on a grand scale (Bell 1989). He acknowledged that a significant number of patients referred to him had personality disorders. He saw incompetent, or even deliberately misleading, expert evidence as a serious problem (Bell 1986).

In 1987 Peter Black published an analysis of 25 consecutive referrals for medicolegal assessment. Without going into reasons, he diagnosed them by the categories of the DSM-III. Of the 25 patients, 13 were depressed, with clinical features conforming with dysthymic disorder, that is neurotic depression, while the symptoms of the others were consistent with adjustment disorder with depressed mood, that being reactive unhappiness. Twelve subjects met DSM-III criteria for conversion disorder, hysterical reaction with *la belle indifférence* and anaesthesias of non-anatomical distribution. Interpersonal difficulties were said to be common.

In general, psychiatrists diagnosed either functional disorder or functional overlay to account for non-organic symptoms. Few thought to raise the issue of causation in legal cases where the employer was being sued for causing a physical injury then. If RSI was not an injury, then causation by mental events, by false beliefs, could be raised in the defence of the claim.

GENERAL PRACTITIONERS AND PRIMARY CARE

Some doctors reported that they held the epidemic at bay. One Canberra practitioner claimed to have raised interest in moral and ethical questions in her first consultations and found that her patients did not go on to develop chronic illness behaviour and soon forgot about their symptoms.

OCCUPATIONAL HEALTH SPECIALISTS

The 1987 edition of *Hunter's Diseases of Occupations* adopted the views of the Australians. Employers were forced to take advice from specialists in occupational health in order to conduct the 'medical surveys' whose protocols were never elucidated.

Dr Malcolm Harrington, Professor of Occupational Health, and Dr Paul Baker, Professor of Rheumatology, at Birmingham University reported on patients they saw as having 'end-stage OOS, occupational overuse syndrome'. At one end of their spectrum of six poultry pluckers were those with symptoms restricted to a single hand tendon that resolved with rest. At the other end was a patient who was so severely affected by what she believed to be overuse that she had to be helped into the consulting room by solicitous relations and who, on examination, was effectively quadriplegic. Both of these patients had performed similar work and one had progressed to a state of invalidity. In Harrington and Baker's analysis:

> In both it was patently obvious that the exacerbating cause was excessive repetitive movements leading to tendonitis which, following prolonged pain and further discomfort had, in the extreme case, led to postural modification, further pain and a progression of symptoms up to and including the shoulder girdle *bilaterally*. Clearly a case of end-stage OOS. (cited in Quintner & Elvey 1991)

Occupational health specialists and occupational therapists' interventions supported their patients' notions concerning both their impairment and their status as disabled. Some advised how work could be divided up into short periods and how it could be done slowly; others advised on gadgets that provided leverage for turning domestic taps.

REHABILITATION SPECIALISTS

The management of RSI became the focus of rehabilitation specialists. Legislation in New South Wales prescribed that a multidisciplinary approach be taken to rehabilitation and a physiotherapist had to be included in any registered rehabilitation centre. Workers were often removed from the workplace to undergo courses in rehabilitation simply because they had reported symptoms.

The fact that psychogenic disorders did not respond to physiotherapy and did not respond to it or other physical remedies escaped the rehabilitation bureaucracy, which was largely composed of physiotherapists.

SURGEONS

Claimants were willing recipients of surgical intervention. No one could believe that a patient was malingering after she had submitted to surgery.

Regulations govern the use of medicines and the government allows their introduction only after clinical trials have determined their efficacy and adverse effects. No trials are required before any new surgical remedy is permitted. Physiotherapy and massage have few risks. In surgery there is an anaesthetic and there are complications, and one of these is that the patient whose symptoms do not respond perceives herself as incurable.

Half of the claimants in my entire sample believed their condition was called carpal tunnel syndrome yet they expected no success from surgery. Ten per cent had surgery without success.

Transplanting the ulnar nerve across its groove was common and this procedure was sometimes offered after carpal tunnel release (CTR) had failed. Occasionally the double diagnosis of concurrent median and ulnar nerve compromise was made to account for symptoms that covered the hand like a glove. Glove distribution is pathognomonic of hysteria. No other condition presents that way. The hypothetical compromise of two nerves at widely separated sites was improbable. How connective tissues at both wrist and elbow could have been affected by an occupational task remained unexamined. Occasionally, radial nerve entrapment was diagnosed in Australia, but this surgery was not popular as it was in the United Kingdom, where one surgeon saw radial nerve entrapment to be a major problem in the RSI stream. How it might have been caused by work remained unexplained.

In the mid-1980s, some doctors in Australia were undertaking a procedure involving hammering the muscles around the epicondyle to traumatise them as a treatment for epicondylitis. That procedure seemed to yield disastrous results.

There was a brief vogue for removal of the first rib. Two separate centres became involved in some sort of surgical manipulation of the brachial plexus, on the basis that posture at work had somehow caused it to be crushed or tangled. One surgeon claimed to have found a dozen or more cases of pisiform necrosis, which he treated surgically to his own satisfaction, but many of his patients remained incapacitated for work. The pisiform is a very small bone in the hand.

Some doctors operated at the wrist to separate, or strip, tendons said to be adhering to each other consequent on chronic tenosynovitis. They reported inflammation of tendons visible to the naked eye but they never offered pathological data to support their observations. Many subjects reported that they had been operated on at the de Quervain's spot at the wrist, but I saw only one correctly diagnosed and successfully treated and that subject had said that typing did not hurt. Scans involving radioactive isotopes later showed activity at former operation sites.

Michael Patkin, a surgeon from Whyalla in South Australia, became an ergonomist and took the position that overuse could only be due to 'abnormal susceptibility or abnormal strain' in a mechanical model. He denounced the idea of labelling it nerves, as he believed 'that 30 per cent of patients attending general practitioners were basically neurotic' (Patkin 1985).

Earl Owen, a microsurgeon, disagreed with the neural hypothesis and took the position that he was dealing with a disease caused by cellular damage that led to unco-ordinated activity of single muscle fibres (Owen 1985). His explanation for different physicians seeing different things was that they saw sufferers whose condition was in different stages of disorganisation.

Hunter Fry, a plastic and facio-maxillary surgeon from Victoria who had 16 refereed publications, published a dozen or more papers about RSI and pain in musicians.

He reported that 'over use injury, (or RSI) has been around since Shakespeare's day'. Fry criticised the notion that RSI was Gowers' occupational neurosis on the grounds that neurosis did not mean the same to Gowers as it does today (Fry 1995, 1996). In this he was correct, as Gowers' concept of neurosis referred to undiagnosable somatic symptoms, whereas today's refers to their emotional causes. Fry's reading of the literature of musicians' cramp failed to reveal that it had psychiatric causes. Again he was not incorrect, as psychogenesis does not imply psychiatric disorder but rather symptoms caused by ideas. In a study of 379 musicians with what he called painful overuse syndrome, Fry reported that RSI appeared to be a distinct clinical entity rather than a collection of unrelated disorders. The patients showed muscular and joint capsule overuse. In his sample, pain generally started in a particular area, then spread both proximally and distally. The patients felt depressed. The treatment was radical rest of the tender structures by the total avoidance of pain-inducing activities.

Fry did not define his terms but he believed that the prevention of overuse lay in the control of use. In another paper, he reported on 612 patients whom he had examined at least once and in whom he had diagnosed RSI in five grades of severity. The ACTU had used the same five-grade classification.

In conjunction with a pathologist, Xenia Dennett, Hunter Fry published a study of biopsies of interosseous muscles of 29 women with painful chronic overuse syndrome and 8 controls in *The Lancet*.

Peter Brooks pointed out that Fry's study had extensive media coverage. He asked:

How can Dennett & Fry state in summary that differences were found when the data show clearly that statistical differences were not found? ... Fry's grading system has not been validated and I was surprised by the choice of muscle that was taken for biopsy since it is the forearm muscles that are more commonly painful in this condition. ... I would hope that the data which show no significant differences in the properly controlled sub-set of patients with bilateral biopsies are the results that are discussed, rather than the incorrect summary. (Brooks 1988)

Bruce Hocking (then Medical Director of Telecom Australia) wrote '[Fry's] findings were based on muscles which had rarely been examined and were seldom the subject of complaint' (Hocking 1988).

Semple, Behan and Behan wrote to the editor:

We find it remarkable that Fry had collected 29 patients with localised pain and tenderness over the first dorsal interosseous muscle, present for more than a year in most of them. ... The danger is that the danger that courts in Australia and elsewhere, might be persuaded by that a real and specific pathological condition existed in patients who merely have complaints rather than clearly identifiable objective physical findings (Semple, Behan and Behan 1988).

Professor Jerzy Sikorski (1985–86) found it a mystery how something he believed to be a 'simple orthopaedic condition has assumed the character of a national crisis, rivalled only by AIDS as a threat to the fabric of our society'. Sikorski found orthopaedic conditions in about half of those whom he saw but he did not detail if the symptoms of which the subjects complained were consistent with the conditions he had diagnosed. He saw the problem in medical, industrial and social terms and thought that the sufferers had not had enough rest.

Ergonomists were called in to ease assumed discomfort and were also paid for providing evaluations of workstations. Some were engineers who had been involved in production techniques; others were physiotherapists with no training for the rapidly expanding work and no knowledge of medicine (Howie & Wyatt 1985).

For the opposition, Bernard Bloch, a surgeon and experienced medicolegal examiner whose opinion had been disregarded in *Lashford v Plessey*, took a sociological viewpoint when he wrote, on the basis of that experience, that 'RSI was a figment of vested interests and politics rather than a medical entity' (Bloch 1984).

Michael Morris and Alan Sharp, surgeons, summarised the characteristics of a non-diagnosis of RSI. They invoked Meador (1965), who had originally used the term 'non-disease'. RSI was characterised by vague, variable and inconsistent symptoms. They could not make any recognisable diagnosis and it progressed despite removal of the alleged cause. Objective physical signs were absent, there were no radiological or serological abnormalities and it only occurred in a compensable context (Morris & Sharp 1985).

Campbell Semple, a distinguished Scottish hand surgeon with particular expertise in brachial plexus surgery, took the view that Quintner and Elvey had been highly selective in the sources from which they built their hypothesis and had used extremes of movement to elicit pain. In his view (1988), Elvey's tests had no established place in diagnosis; the brachial plexus and its branches could accommodate the vast majority of movements.

PHYSIOTHERAPISTS

In general, physiotherapists were followers of the injury paradigm and they delivered physical remedies. Some medical practitioners appropriated physiotherapeutic remedies and purchased laser machines, ultrasound generators and acupuncture equipment and delivered the treatments themselves. The availability of these remedies was advertised in large lettering on shopfront surgeries.

Most treatment practices were recycled, in that they had been tried a century earlier and had been reported as unsuccessful in the treatment of writers' cramp. The vast majority of treatments offered could be passively received: ultrasound and neck traction, massage, wax baths, laser therapy, exercises, soft collars, bandages, lotions, ointments and sprays, galvanic and transcutaneous electrical nerve stimulation (TENS). Physiotherapeutic remedies were not without attendant risks. Ultrasound almost universally made functional symptoms worse; ice baths carried the risk of thermal injury; neck traction caused permanent complications in several patients whom I interviewed.

I made several attempts to obtain reports from the manufacturers of laser therapy machines to learn how they worked and how they had been tested. The manufacturers supplied glossy pamphlets and price lists, but literature on clinical trials was never made available.

Acupuncture was not limited to Chinese-trained therapists. The claimants whom I had examined conceded no success to the many lotions, ointments, sprays and bandages, which were in vogue. Virtually every remedy undertaken helped at the time, but the symptoms returned very soon after.

THEORETICAL MEDICINE

Anthony Lowy (1983, 1984) held that RSI suggested autonomic nervous system dysfunction but remained well aware of a role for psychological factors.

MEDICAL JOURNALS

The medical literature in refereed journals cited in this book failed to retrieve the origins of both the name and the concept of RSI. The legitimation of cause by the NHMRC had provided the major reference of authority. The activities of unions in circulating information and facilitating the process of claiming passed unremarked. Little, if any, comment was made in the medical press concerning the circulation of the multitude of pamphlets on prevention of RSI and the role played by the guides to diagnosis in suggesting symptomatology.

The editor of the *Medical Journal of Australia* declined to tell me when I asked if these papers had been subjected to independent refereeing procedures.

The original proponents of the injury theory issued no retractions, nor did the *Medical Journal of Australia*. The 1987 papers, under the editorial of Professor David Ferguson, challenged the injury theory, but their publication did not have much benefit for the claimants who were already afflicted (Ferguson 1987; Wright 1987, Cleland 1987).

Ferguson was the only one of the initial injury theorists to declare his change of heart. His original position underpinned a case *Abalos v the Australian Postal Commission*, which reached the High Court in 1990. That case was decided on the basis of expert evidence that Ferguson had, by that time, repudiated.

Between 1988 and 1991, the *Medical Journal of Australia* closed correspondence on RSI. The debate then continued into 1993, with the parties remaining entrenched in their respective positions. While agreement was reached that RSI was not a good name for the condition, little concession was made to the possibility that the symptoms represented somatization and that their causes were ideas and emotions.

PSYCHOLOGISTS

The most comprehensive explanations came from academic psychologists. Those in a treatment role would have been excluded from managing clients if they openly espoused a psychological explanation.

Professional psychologists were well aware of the scope of somatization and illness behaviour, but those working in occupational health clinics came under medical dominance and under the same influences as the medical profession. Some offered stress management and pain management techniques. All personal difficulties were attributed to RSI and this effectively prevented claimants from taking responsibility for their symptoms. The secondary gain of having time to attend to children, sick parents and other competing responsibilities was either ignored or not recognised.

If patients were not conceptualised as having an injury caused by work, the psychologist could not claim fees from an insurer. Perception of symptoms through a somatization model threatened the receipt of compensation and, by extension, the claiming of fees for treating it. Psychologists seeking fees in private practice faced the market; there were no health insurance fund rebates for psychological therapies.

Academic psychologists who had no interest in treatment took other views. Robert Spillane, Professor in the School of Management at Macquarie University, argued that RSI was an industrial issue brought about by changes in behaviour and attitudes to symptoms in the workplace and that this had brought about medicalisation. He considered the decision to take certain action in regard to symptoms to be a moral choice and passed no judgment on it. Rather, Spillane predicted that society would need to decide whether people with pain in the absence of diagnosable disease should be compensated as patients or treated as autonomous working people communicating various dissatisfactions. Spillane and Deves questioned whether RSI was 'pretence or patienthood' or 'a social movement' or 'a consequence of the dogmatism of those who sought to reduce human problems to medical theology' (Spillane & Deves 1986, 1987; Deves & Spillane 1989).

In 1988, Professor Wayne Hall and Louise Morrow published a paper that stressed that the epidemiology of RSI was inconsistent with a notion that it was an injury caused by repetitive movements or extended static loading in the workplace. They identified the reasons for endemic symptoms producing substantial disability when they came to media and public attention. They recognised the role of the occupational health and safety movement, the use of workers' health issues to improve working conditions, the fact that RSI appeared when a new technology was being blamed for increasing unemployment, the newspaper and media coverage and the contagion in the workplace exacerbated by the wide acceptance of the compensable status of workplace symptoms.

The incidence of RSI actually rose at a time employment was improving from a trough in 1983, to a peak in 1984. The economy was characterised by change that involved a transfer of jobs from the manufacturing to the services sector.

Hall and Morrow identified factors promoting disability: the iatrogenic process which included the medicolegal system, over-concern on the part of the patients' doctors, methods of medical management predisposing to disability, the attribution of cause to the work environment, the hope of receiving gain through the legal system and to having to demonstrate illness or disability for the duration of the litigation process.

MEDICAL FORMULATIONS

Claimants expressed themselves in medical-sounding terms and reported having received any number between one and 14, with an average of more than six, of the following diagnoses: algodynia, algodystrophy, arthritis, carpal tunnel syndrome, causalgia, curvature of the spine, de Quervain's tenosynovitis, epicondylitis, extensor tenosynovitis, flexor tenosynovitis, frozen shoulder, Gerhardt's knuckle syndrome, inflammation, intersection syndrome, lateral epicondylitis, lumps, medial epicondylitis, mild tennis elbow, nerves not conducting, neck or muscle overuse, pisiform necrosis, problems (including bulges) at any of the cervical discs, radial nerve entrapment, Raynaud's disease, reflex sympathetic dystrophy, regional pain syndrome, RSI, Scheuremann's osteochondritis, strained muscles, sympathetic dystrophy, tangled brachial plexus, tendonitis in multiple locations, tenosynovitis, tension neck, thoracic outlet syndrome and having an ulnar or a radial nerve which needed to be relocated.

Not only were there no curbs on private medicine in Australia, there was also no concept of over-servicing in workers' compensation. Such entrepreneurial activities were positively encouraged in this epidemic and prestigious government institutions, including teaching hospitals, indulged in them. Such medical practices do not come under scrutiny when costs of workers' compensation blow out. Inevitably, the government tried to remove lawyers, but did not try to control doctors in a later scheme. Courts never did make an order that an insurer need not reimburse a treatment or an investigation, even if they were manifestly useless; this potential for constraint was simply never invoked. Seriously injured patients got less money, but useless remedies continued to be indemnified.

UNIONS AND INSTITUTIONS

The ACTU took its advice from those doctors whose views had been legitimated by the NHMRC, the same ones who advised the Task Force into RSI in the Australian Public Service and the National Occupational Health and Safety Commission.

The Standards Association of Australia, at the request of the Human Factors Committee of the Safety Standards Board, was engaged to prepare a proposal on the prevention, and it called for submissions. No report emerged. The Safety Institute of Australia held seminars in conjunction with physiotherapists to teach skills of RSI management.

Other commercial enterprises promoted gadgets and gimmicks, selling pads on which typewriters might be placed, wrist splints of many kinds, laser generating machines for use in skin stimulation and ointments to ease the pain. A cream was repeatedly advertised on the radio as helpful in RSI cases. Publications purporting to explain RSI were sold in health food stores and chemist shops and by mail order. Guides for the self-help movement included *RSI: An Explorer's Guidebook* (Brennan 1985) and *RSI Explained* (Arndt 1986).

Apple advertised its split NORSI keyboard with the phrase 'no RSI' and warned of RSI in its manuals. 'Microsoft draws your attention to a word most word processing software doesn't want to know about, tenosynovitis' appeared throughout 1986 in a series of advertisements in weekend colour supplements.

SOCIOLOGISTS

Evan Willis was struck in 1986 by the absence of sociological comment on what he saw as a tantalising subject. He compared the use of RSI in mediating industrial relations with the use of miners' nystagmus, which developed in England and Wales at times of threatened mine closures and increased union activity. Nystagmus is a condition in which the eyes flicked if one looked sideways, and it had also been classified as an occupational neurosis. The epidemiology of miners' nystagmus failed to correlate its onset with any aspect of mining, other than the threatened closure of mines and exacerbations of industrial conflict. Compensation was paid for this epidemic disorder (Figlio 1982).

In 1989 Dr Anthony Hopkins, a sociologist, published a paper in the *Australian and New Zealand Journal of Sociology*. This paper read like a personal attack on me. I was mentioned by name or by pronoun 13 times in nine paragraphs, which contained no fewer than eight serious misquotes. He accused me of producing 'a serious distortion of the past' in my 'analysis of nineteenth and early twentieth century arm pain epidemics' and of taking 'essentially a non-scientific approach' ('her epistemology is akin to that of a religious believer') and finally writing that 'anyone who could seriously expect feminists to be persuaded by this argument needs to see a psychiatrist!'

FEMINISTS

Some feminists perceived RSI as a consequence of the exploitation of women by men and protested vociferously against the diagnosis of somatization (for example, Turner 1984; Meekosha 1986). They construed the sufferers as victims and debunked a diagnosis of psychogenic disorder as dismissive. Meekosha was shrewd and observant when she saw psychiatrists asking: 'Can these women be made to come to terms with their true role in society, their true female functions and these, of course, are assumed to revolve around child bearing and child rearing: the woman as a reproductive and nurturing machine?'

Meekosha correctly identified the numerous conflicts experienced by women. However, she underestimated the extent to which many of them were faced with a choice between working and attending to those same responsibilities. Meekosha argued her case with sophistication, citing Freud's mismanagement of the case of Dora. With less sophistication, she attributed bad faith to doctors, alleging that they only diagnosed a neurotic condition in an attempt to disguise their inability to cure.

It was my view, on the basis of what I was seeing, that women had more RSI than did men, because women had more obligations conflicting with their responsibilities at work.

Denise Russell (1988a), a philosopher, rejected the argument for somatization, asserting, but not demonstrating, that there were empirical grounds for doing so. She launched an attack on me in the *Journal of Community Health Studies*, in which she claimed that evidence was accumulating for the physical causation of RSI. She charged that I held my views for profit and she believed that they were detrimental to the health of RSI sufferers.

Russell argued through a series of misquotes, misconstruals and personal insults, attributing to me ideas that had been neither expressed nor intended (Russell 1988b). She failed to reveal the grounds on which she had based them. Her attempts at debunking were based on her assumption that the injury theory was well substantiated scientifically. There was little philosophical discussion in her work.

THE PERCEPTIONS OF THE CLAIMANTS

Claimants were assessed by up to a dozen experts, each of whom tended to see RSI in terms of diagnoses and remedies available within his or her expertise.

Claimants quickly learnt from published guides and medical examinations how their symptoms should be reported, what issues attracted the attention of doctors, what symptoms were interesting to doctors and what were and were not acceptable attribution theories. In one medical practice, guides to the identification of RSI were left among magazines in the waiting room. The doctor then checked off the patients' symptoms from a list. Having passed this viva voce, the patients were told that they really did have RSI, and RSI duly appeared on their medical certificates.

Self-help groups were formed 'for the purposes of monitoring developments in the field of RSI, for research and for recruitment of appropriate medical and legal advisers'. These were funded by union money as well as by direct grants from government instrumentalities (McIntosh 1986). The volunteer workers for an organisation called Women's Repetitive Injury Support Team (WRIST) complained that they had been given a research grant of only $70 000 from the Victorian government when they had asked for $200 000.

The afflicted workers sought legitimation of their suffering as real, physical and caused by work. They responded to the availability of therapeutic relationships, which in turn exposed them to the possibility of being exploited and to remedies that were unlikely to ameliorate symptoms. Attribution theories were hard to separate from medical words posing as diagnostic labels. When a person believed that her pain was called epicondylitis, de Quervain's syndrome, frozen shoulder or any other condition known to have a traumatic origin, there was no further inquiry demanded. The cause was assumed to be occupational.

Each worker identified a breach in union-promoted workplace standards and reported it to her physician. New cramp subjects developed newer attribution theories to accommodate their situations.

As information spread, RSI emerged in workplaces that had been the same for years. Some blamed chairs of the wrong height, badly positioned VDUs, faulty work stations, old typewriters, poorly designed furniture, inactivity, incorrect posture, badly designed equipment and furniture. This last group cited the opinions of furniture manufacturers, salesmen and ergonomists to support their case. A handful cited noise, and appeared irritated when they were asked how exposure to noise could account for arm pain or how equipment, posture or furniture could be responsible for symptoms years later.

Some claimants attributed their problems to use, to overuse, to not having enough to do or, paradoxically, having too much to do in the sense of having an endless supply of work. Some saw themselves as being allergic to the keyboard; others attributed their problem to the position in which they had held their hands.

Many attributed their problems to new keyboards attached to word-processing equipment. The common soft touch keyboard was feared in some circles in Canberra. Some government departments had to re-equip themselves with technology approved by unions and were forced to discard those computers the unions had demonised (RSI Task Force 1984). There was some uncertain blaming of multinational firms who were said to have dumped inferior equipment on the Australian market and these ideas were fuelled by reports of successful litigation against various computer companies (Kavanagh 1984). Some blamed specific brands, but no brand emerged as more blamed than any other.

One woman returned from overseas and became affected. Recognising that there were no physical differences between her workplace abroad and the one in Australia and, recognising the sheer absurdity of the prevalent attribution theories, she suggested that Black Mountain tower, a microwave transmission facility overlooking Canberra, was the cause of the local epidemic. Her doctor documented that, in his opinion, she suffered from delusions and he continued to promote his various keyboard theories.

Claims were legitimated by medical practitioners on the basis that a person had worked too fast or too slowly or too repetitively or simply for too many years and just felt worn out. Claims were made on the basis that a footrest had not been provided and that chairs and tables had been of the wrong height and that a short person had to sit on telephone books to bring her into a comfortable position.

In factories, medical advisers attributed RSI to 'having done the same thing for too long' and, paradoxically, 'to being unaccustomed to the task'. Some blamed a machine which worked too fast, others blamed having to perform forceful movements and the demands that quotas be met, while others attributed their problems to not having enough to do. Disliked supervisors got their share of blame.

The rest, finding no fault in their work situation, simply argued: 'It must have been work, as I did not have it before and I have it now'.

THE SOCIAL HISTORY OF AFFLICTED CLAIMANTS

A social history of RSI patients was documented in detail by Reid and others and by Eva Lowy in a doctoral dissertation. They interviewed 52 women from a chicken processing plant and from a telecommunications agency, describing what they called the 'the pilgrimage of pain', that is, the search for legitimation. They recognised that the women were expressing their dissatisfactions with working conditions and that they saw them as dangerous to their health.

Their conclusion was that the failure of the dominant explanations for RSI contributed to their chronicity. This group spurned the diagnosis of occupational neurosis for what they called its 'logical flaws', but they did not detail what these were.

About half of their sample were still employed at the time of the interview and were continuing to work in pain. They had gone through the processes of symptom evaluation, then illness action then, finally, adaptation to being sick. In the area of illness action, the women described months or years of doctor shopping, with forays into the world of alternative medicine. While some doctors diagnosed their symptoms in the sense of giving them a name and a prognosis, they felt that other doctors did not know how to help them. The response of the doctors was said to have ranged from bewildered to frankly sceptical. They reported that their doctors did not know much about RSI until they gave them papers and union documents.

With these women, the doctor did not need to be knowledgeable to be praised. The object of desire was to be believed, to have one's suffering legitimated as physical and compensable. Thirty-three per cent of this group changed their doctors, some as many as three times, in their pursuit of one who knew about RSI and was sympathetic. The treatments offered by non-medical health professionals were equally ineffective in the long term; some women said that they were 'a complete waste of time'. While the women's experiences with practitioners of alternative medicine were almost always positive, they spoke well of medical practitioners who had told them that there was nothing they could do. They were informed that the problem was work related, that they would never do clerical work again, that they probably would never be completely rid of the condition and not to expect any miracles because the damage had been done.

Others were told that the splints they had worn had permanently wasted the muscles in their arms and, if they did not rest further, they would become crippled. Seventy-eight per cent of women had been told to rest.

The affected women were apparently predisposed to the very biases of which they complained in doctors and they were reluctant to accept that the distress and disability of others was genuine. In the view of these affected subjects, there were two categories of claimants: the 'liars, bunging it on, out to get what they could out of the company' and 'genuine cases' like their own.

The women found the insurance-nominated doctors to be widely scattered geographically and their interpretations of the interviews with them were less than charitable and in some cases frankly disingenuous.

Lowy did not set out to challenge the women's views of themselves or their condition, but dealt with the women's perceptions and experiences. No attempts were made to see the problems as responses to stress or conflict in the women's lives, all of which remained unexamined.

THE MEDIA

The media were responsible for publicising RSI, and their role cannot be overestimated. Before December 1983, when the first paper about RSI appeared in the medical press, there were 3000 cases in the Australian Public Service and the phenomenon was being reported in the popular press (Smith 1982). Information travelled from the media to patient, then from patient to the doctor. This form of transmission of medical information in the case of psychosomatic disorders has been documented by Shorter (1992), who noted that the patients' paradigm preceded the doctors' paradigm and changed ahead of it.

RSI was the most commonly mentioned issue in the press in 1985. Most articles were based on the press releases of the ACTU. RSI and the Workers' Health Centre were incorporated into an episode of the long-running television soap opera, *A Country Practice*.

On the subject of carpal tunnel syndrome as a consequence of work, Dr Mac, a regular columnist, wrote in the *Sunday Telegraph*:

> Carpal tunnel syndrome is one of the conditions of the joints, bones, tendons and muscles that may be related to RSI. ... If you use your wrist a great deal, as in typing or playing the piano, the tendons may become strained and inflamed. ... Treatment should be sought at the first sign of a pain in the hand or wrist, not when the pain becomes unbearable. (29 April 1991)

This implies that symptoms that are reminiscent or suggestive of a clinical condition can be managed as if they are that condition. Publication of symptom lists encouraged vulnerable individuals, worried about their health, to identify themselves as afflicted. The medical journalist can omit essential elements, such as negating or superfluous symptoms of a kind that can only be elicited by a skilled diagnostician.

Journalists and union research officers made numerous educational videos. Audiovisual materials were shown in workplaces at lunch breaks and during union meetings. One video produced by Channel 10 showed a hand in a state of apparent paralysis and declared it to be in 'stage III' of RSI. This was promoted as the outcome if early warning symptoms were ignored. This video caused some workers to 'realise' the 'true' meaning of sensations they had previously regarded as tiredness or discomfort. Insurance companies noted that cases of RSI came forward from each workplace within days of this video being shown (Dr A Christie, GIO, pers. com.).

Journalists attributed RSI to a variety of social forces and pathogenic agents. When physicians or experts figured in the popular press, it was generally because they had some theory to account for the epidemic or a new idea concerning the pathology of the disorder.

Anti-fluoridationists suspected that RSI was a long-term consequence of the drinking of fluoridated water. Dentists disagreed with them.

Auberon Waugh wrote in *The Spectator*, in November 1986, 'Introducing Kangaroo's Paw, a wonderful new disease from Australia'. His joke was that if you slept with a woman you got a baby, if you slept with a man you got AIDS and if you slept alone you got RSI. He prophesied a tremendous future for what he called this 'wankers' disease' in Britain.

Anna-Maria Dell'Oso reported a brush with arm pain in 1986, while 'tracking down an elusive sentence in the thick undergrowth of the word forest'. In analysing her options, she reported on the lives of friends, forever explaining themselves to relatives, doctors, psychologists, bosses, union officials, solicitors and government bureaucrats. She observed it among the more conscientious workers. 'The battle,' she wrote, 'was fought out under the banners of body, mind, drugs, knife or analysis.' She found it tempting to dutifully put her paws into splints and think no more about it until the next nervous breakdown. She was influenced by the Alexander technique and the 'thing' left her. She asked, 'Why must we split ourselves up like that?'

The *Australian Women's Weekly* (March 1985) cited the *Status of Women Report* and advised its readers to divide long household activities into shorter periods.

THE COMMUNITY

The beliefs of the community about the epidemic reflected medical explanations, social tensions and the beliefs that healers of all persuasions held about the disorder. Their beliefs were governed by their acculturation, education and wishes to be involved, especially where that involvement was related to their interests.

10

CONCLUSION: EXPERT EVIDENCE, MEDICINE AND THE LAW

> The history of Lysenko is finished. The history of the
> causes of Lysenkoism continues. One History is at
> an end. Is the other endless?
>
> Louis Althusser

Like Freidson, I do not wish to overlook medical advancements. I do not seek to undermine the professional services of physicians, the vast majority of which are carried out with care and competence. The problem of which I have written was created by individuals who placed their own idiosyncratic beliefs on a higher level than the existing body of medical knowledge.

History tells us that physicians are likely to be influential beyond their capabilities when they become moral entrepreneurs and lend their expertise to the state, in pursuit of goals serving a moral imperative, one which they place higher than their own training as clinicians in orthodox medicine. When power, rather than science, supports them, they are easily captured by the reality of their social constructions.

A society can have any kind of workers' compensation scheme it wants, but industry has to be capable of funding it. No country can fund a system based on incorrect, that is, false, concepts of causation.

When Professor Ferguson supported RSI as a disease caused by some general aspect of working conditions in *Abalos v The Australian Postal Commission* (Supreme Court of New South Wales 1987), he gave evidence that he was 'appalled' at what he considered to be the inhuman production line operations in the coding room. He stated that, simply from an inspection of the work, it was quite foreseeable 'that at least a proportion of the operators would suffer ... damage ... including the generalised muscle injury called RSI'. The Court of Appeal reversed the decision that the Australian Postal Commission had been negligent.

Abalos appealed successfully and, by the time the case reached the High Court, Professor Ferguson had effectively abandoned his beliefs about RSI being an injury of any kind, let alone one negligently caused (Ferguson 1987).

The ability to evaluate science in expert evidence is still a scarce resource, but education in this needs to increase and courses in judging science and evidence should be available for the judiciary. Judges see themselves as being under no obligation, legal or moral, to give consideration to the unintended consequences of their actions, provided that the decisions have been made within the framework of the law.

It is reasonable to suspect that judges and juries resonate with the invalid beliefs held by the rest of the community. Judges may cite precedent or may even feel an obligation to adhere to the common views of a society. Courts provide legitimation. They serve as unwitting corroborators of the community's beliefs. Courts have the power to determine what is factual and this is precisely what they do. They do not, however, do this in a way that distinguishes what the law constructs as a fact from what is the case in scientific knowledge.

Judicial decisions sometimes legitimate false causes. These, in turn, cause the adoption of time-consuming, expensive, wasteful and defensive procedures. Judicial decisions can create new medical categories, from nervous shock to RSI. Rather than evaluate testimony, judges and juries may chose to adopt the view of the expert who allows them to make the decision that they want to make, one that seems to suit society's needs, the needs of the individual claimant or what they see as the public good. Failure of the judiciary to understand hysteria has caused, and continues to cause, many tragedies.

In 1643, against a background of the Inquisition in France, the Abbé Grandier, a priest in Loudon, was accused by a group or Ursuline nuns of coming at night, as an incubus, to have sexual congress with them. The ecclesiastical courts of the time convicted him on the nuns' accusations and he was punished by execution. In today's language, the Abbé was convicted on the content of the hysterical beliefs of the nuns and not because he had done it. The experts of the time were unable or unwilling to tell the difference between the belief and the actual state of affairs. It is still the case today that courts do not differentiate from beliefs and actualities.

We wish to believe that our experts and our courts have a better theoretical framework within which to operate than they did 350 years ago. We would like to think that our own beliefs at the start of the twenty-first century are better and have been better evaluated than were the beliefs prevalent in the seventeenth century. Yet we continue to have moral panics, driven by junk science and the tabloid media.

The courts regularly fail now, as they did then, to distinguish false, fashionable beliefs from those held on a solid scientific basis.

Courts still convict innocent people, organisations and processes when they attribute false cause to an event. Courts penalise and punish the convicted on evidence that can be utterly and completely wrong. A conviction of an individual or an institution is not just when it is based on pseudo-science, on hysterical beliefs that drive whatever is the current moral panic. There can be no justice based on falsehood. The responsibility of the courts to differentiate hysterical attribution theories from scientifically validated causes still needs to be addressed in Australia.

In the United States, the decision in *Daubert v Merrell Dow Pharmaceuticals* (Supreme Court of the United States 1993) differentiated the opinions of experts from expert evidence and this process has been incorporated into American federal law. The unanimous ruling states that the criterion of the scientific status of a proposition is that is can be tested, particularly by way of a logical process called falsification. That is, it must be possible to specify a set of circumstances, the occurrence of which would demonstrate that the proposition is false if it is false.

In effect, *Daubert* replaces the *Frye* (1923) and *Bolam* (1923) tests of expert opinion, being that which is generally accepted by a significant number of authorities in the field, with Karl Popper's notion of science as knowledge that has withstood rigorous testing. This sometimes entails a preliminary assessment, a Daubert hearing, to decide if the reasoning or methodology underlying the testimony is scientifically valid. However, it seems that laws can be made on junk science assumptions that would not pass a Daubert hearing. I refer to legal definitions of carpal tunnel syndrome or cumulative trauma disorders in some of the United States.

Daubert has not been adopted in Australia, where simple plausibility of expertise still holds sway, with *Abalos* (High Court of Australia 1990) and *Adamcik* (High Court of Australia 1961) setting the standard. Adamcik, a tram conductor, had tortiously sustained injuries in the course of his work and, a few weeks after his discharge from hospital, he had developed leukaemia and died. His widow sued. The mainstream of medical evidence was that leukaemia was a disease of the white blood cells, in which they reproduced themselves to an abnormal degree, and its origin was in the chromosomes of the affected cells. Nonetheless, a physician of some age and dignity was found who was of the opinion that the physical injuries sustained, together with the accompanying mental stress, had caused the leukaemia. It was apparent that his opinion was not supported by scientific or statistical information. He was the only medical practitioner known to hold that opinion. The jury accepted his evidence and the widow won her right to lifelong compensation. The Government Transport Commissioner appealed to the High Court. The judge seemed to pass up an opportunity to define what constituted expert evidence and to differentiate it legally from those offerings that were no more than the opinions of experts. Rather, he reaffirmed the right of the jury to choose the expert it preferred. In *Abalos,* the High Court gave the judge the same right to judge, if he wished, an expert witness by his demeanour. My legal colleagues informed me that this is the law, this is correct, this is what judges and juries have the power to do and that I would be well advised to forget my intellectual pretensions and to concentrate on charm.

Scientific method includes putting up a proposition couched in the negative, a null hypothesis, and testing it to see if it can be knocked down. Examples of the null hypothesis are that the accused is not guilty and that the unicorn does not exist. One can never prove that a unicorn does not exist, as it might always be just out of sight, so a proposition asserting that a unicorn exists is not a suitable one for a scientific investigation. The presumption of innocence is a null hypothesis, a hallmark of good law as well as good science. In junk science, the null hypothesis is replaced by a positive assertion, one that cannot be proved to be untrue even if it is untrue.

Karl Popper would say that the proposition that RSI is an injury is not one suitable for scientific investigation. If scientific criteria ruled expert evidence, it would no longer be acceptable for a person with the status of an expert to argue that one cannot prove that RSI, whatever it is, is not caused by work. It remains to be seen what will come of the RSI epidemic in the United States if the injury of RSI is ever subjected to a Daubert hearing.

I dedicate this book to all those who have suffered as a consequence of junk science and hysterical beliefs.

11

RSI: 'A BLESSING IN DISGUISE'

All names have been changed and these cases are given names in alphabetical order. No cramp subject can be identified from these histories.

This is the case study that gave this chapter its name, number 55:

Miss Smith, a 37-year-old single mother of three, had worked part-time as a VDU operator. She had been absent from work for 14 months and had not returned.

Her doctor, in the course of a consultation on another issue, incidentally told her the computers at work caused all the swelling in her hands. Miss Smith had formerly attributed these to sewing her children's clothes. While receiving compensation, she started to study full-time for her Higher School Certificate, at college from 9:00 till 3:00, three days a week. With unusual frankness, she referred to the diagnosis of RSI as 'a blessing in disguise'. She was concerned with the welfare of her children and had not really wanted to go back to work. Miss Smith continued to receive workers' compensation to supplement her Supporting Mother's Benefit (a category of social security payment) and this brought her income up to more than she could have earned from full-time work. Moreover, she did not have to bear the expenses of going to work, so she was significantly better off. It made no sense to go to work if she could keep more money by staying home, being a student and caring for her children.

TWENTY CASES

The first 20 randomly selected cases are summarised here. This sample was generated from 319 cases seen and reported on between 1986 and 1991. Their files were listed in alphabetical order and the cases selected by number screen.

Information was extracted from claimants' files. The development of symptoms, their multiple diagnoses, treatment-seeking behaviour and the remedies they attracted are documented in counterpoint with their social predicaments.

I created diagnostic categories to improve on the overriding descriptive of 'somatizing'. All, bar three, were somatizing. The formulation 'hysteria/nothing at all' refers, in these cases, to a situation where a conflict was resolved or need was satisfied by sick leave and the person was apparently acting in good faith. No psychiatric diagnosis can be made as there is little, if any, evidence of distress. Seeking a predictable diagnostician could be seen as a culturally approved response to stress at that period, hence hysteria is not, in this context, an illness.

'Disease' refers to a lesion diagnosis without somatoform symptomatology.

'Functional disorder' refers to cases in which palpable anxiety and depression were being experienced emotionally as well as, in part, as symptoms in the body. Some could not be classified as many factors were operating and different factors had operated at other times.

'Functional overlay' refers to cases in which there had been some local pathology, not necessarily related to work; for example, there is no organic lesion that results from typing, but workers in manufacturing did suffer from various arm conditions well described in textbooks of industrial rheumatology, such as that of Nortin Hadler, to which reference has been made. In these patients, symptoms had multiplied, had gone on for too long and had caused more work disability than the original lesion could have done.

'Malingering' referred to people who told lies, behaved dishonestly on physical examination, withheld strategic information or were otherwise inconsistent and deceptive. Some might have somatized earlier in their period of absence but their disability was, to a greater or lesser extent, contrived.

In general, the stresses were age-related. The youngest women were more likely to be in two minds about working because they were having relationships, getting married or having babies. The middle group were more likely to be having problems with children for whom they had to get care during their working hours. Some were getting divorced. The oldest group were more likely to be dealing with deaths or chronic illness in their close families and with their own health problems.

CASE NUMBER 3

Miss Adams was 20-year-old telex operator who had been absent from work for eight months and had not returned. She recited her story word for word from Tenosynovitis Association pamphlets. 'I've got some tendons. Your tendons are in a shaft. You're doing rapid repetitive movements, it just explains what happens. It just dries up.'

Her symptoms had come on with severe shooting pains in both forearms with symmetrical pain symptoms involving her hand, wrist, forearm, elbow, upper arm, shoulder and neck, backs and fronts of both her arms, and pins and needles in the tips of her fingers and on the palmar surfaces of her palms. These symptoms extended and involved the entire top half of her body. Miss Adams claimed that she had lost the use of her arms.

She herself had prescribed and purchased her splints. She consulted several medical and paramedical therapists and she was able to tell me that they attributed her symptoms to RSI, repetitive work, rapid movements, tenosynovitis, inflammation, keyboard work, shoulder, neck and brachial neuralgia.

Miss Adams' arm symptoms had started when she developed a serious relationship with a young man and she took a medical certificate for compensation when she moved to be with him in the country. Her family doctor had told her that she 'kept going down with psychosomatic disorders' and had sent her to a psychiatrist, whom she saw once but refused to see again. In contemptuous terms, she spoke of doctors who 'tell you nothing' while she accepted the construction that the union had put on her symptoms. 'My having RSI made everyone more aware,' she told me, happy to have become a focus of attention.

I could make no diagnosis other than nothing/pure hysteria, or conversion disorder. This might have been part of an overriding tendency to somatize. Miss Adams could not have easily travelled in to work daily from where she was living, as it would have involved a round trip of over three hours.

CASE NUMBER 7

Mrs Brown, a 21-year-old data entry operator, described a painful paralysis in one arm, a palsy which been transient. Although she did not stop work, she had claimed for physiotherapist's bills. She was given a front office job, which she preferred to data input, so she had gained this advantage by complaining. The office joke, she said, had been, 'Get RSI and get yourself some money'. Mrs Brown reported these symptoms just two months after she and her husband had bought a house and incurred a substantial mortgage. Mrs Brown wanted to have a child, but, financially, she was not in a position to do that. I could not see anything other than that she was testing the water to see if she got away with malingering.

CASE NUMBER 9

Mrs Cherub, a 22-year-old process worker, had taken long periods off work over the previous three years on compensation. When I saw her, she was again on compensation and had not worked for five months.

Swelling was experienced on the radial aspect of her wrist and it progressed into the upper arm and neck, with pins and needles in the back of her right hand after work. Her symptoms also involved the backs of her hands.

Mrs Cherub was given a cream, then five weeks on compensation and a change of task in the factory before being moved to clerical work. Painkillers of various kinds made no difference; ultrasound made her worse. She wore a splint that, she said, helped her because when she put it on she did not do so much repetitive work. Not working, rest, electric/galvanic stimulation and changing the grip on her pen were all equally useless. She was treated for RSI, overuse attributed to repetitive work, brachial neuralgia and a neck disc problem.

For the duration of her claim, Mrs Cherub's husband was also receiving compensation following a car accident. Two months after she first went off work and three years before I saw her, she and her husband had bought a house and taken on a substantial mortgage. That same year she bore her first child, and soon after, a second one, both while she was on compensation. Mrs Cherub reported herself as 'separated' in the middle of her pregnancy and she received a supporting parent's benefit from Social Security, as well as compensation. The husband received a substantial settlement, and he bought a taxi and immediately started driving it. When I saw her some months after he received his settlement, she was pregnant with a third child and again on compensation.

Mrs Cherub's claim straddled three employers and three insurers. Her case was riddled with fraud and her presentation was disingenuous. There was a personality problem in evidence and the rest of the formulation was obscure.

CASE NUMBER 11

Mrs Dawson was a 23-year-old stenographer who had gone back to work, having been absent on compensation for nine months. She had to work harder than she liked to do. When she got tired, her doctors medicalised her fatigue, calling it RSI. A medical certificate was issued to the effect that she was not to do more than 15 minutes of typing per hour for no more than four hours a day. This regimen was of no help at all, so she went off work for a month. Her symptoms then moved from left to right and she complained of tired arms and pins and needles.

An occupational therapist's assessment of the workplace resulted in her recommending an adjustable table, a new word processor, an adjustable chair, a footstool, a typewriter and 15-minute rest breaks each hour.

Mrs Dawson tried three types of splints and physiotherapy.

Electric pulse therapy aggravated her symptoms whereas ultrasound was said to have taken the swelling down. She had not noticed any swelling herself, but her doctor, allegedly, had drawn her attention to it. None was in evidence when I saw her. She attended rehabilitation at a workers' health clinic for nine and a half months, building up her attendance there to four days of work a week. Rehabilitation involved craft groups and discussions with other RSI subjects. She later returned to full duties but complained about the furniture. She learnt to attribute her problem to having typed with her wrists in extension. Ice treatments were given three times a week, giving rise to the possibility of thermal injury.

Mrs Dawson took time off after she got tired, and she spoke to a journalist who had come from an organisation that 'knew all about RSI'. During this period, trade union workers were recruiting potential RSI subjects from workplaces and making appointments for them to see doctors in the various workers clinics. She claimed to have the support of her union. Her mother had died suddenly at the age of 43, about 18 months before the onset of the arm symptoms, and Mrs Dawson had married four weeks later. These stressors were not counted in this survey's statistics as neither event was sufficiently close to being seen as a precipitating stress. Strong iatrogenic and political factors seemed to be operating here. I could not classify this case otherwise.

CASE NUMBER 23

Mrs Elissa, a 26-year-old clerk, had been absent from work on compensation for over two years and had returned to work at the time of interview.

Mrs Elissa had attended a doctor with her toddler son, who had a cold. According to her, the doctor incidentally noted a lump on her wrist, commented on it and asked her what work she had been doing. When she told him that she was a data input operator, he diagnosed RSI and told her to go off work for three months.

Mrs Elissa attended a workers' clinic and was unable to get light duties; she was sacked. She then took more than two years off work on compensation, attending to her child and studying at university. She was given further time off on compensation as well as physiotherapy, massage, hot baths, ultrasound, stretching exercises, electric/galvanic stimulation, cortisone injections, nonsteroidal anti-inflammatory drugs, unidentified tablets and acupuncture, all to no avail, although the acupuncture helped her headaches.

Mrs Elissa protested that she liked her work and that she only stopped on her doctor's advice. Her mother, who had been minding her child, had just returned to her country of origin at the time Mrs Elissa started to get certificates. She was seeing a psychiatrist for depression, but by the time I saw her she was working and attending university on their disabled quota to study psychology as part of her rehabilitation.

Mrs Elissa's symptoms had started towards the end of an unhappy and unsatisfactory marriage. She had started to recover after the divorce but she stayed on compensation. She had resolved her conflict between working and caring for the child, but later she became depressed when her marriage ended. Continuing arm pain might have been part of that.

CASE NUMBER 25

Mrs Fritz, a 27-year-old process worker involved in packing boxes, had been absent from work for more than five years and had not returned.

Packing had originally given her a sore thumb, but her symptoms extended to both arms and particularly to her neck. A pain in the wrist went on to symptoms that multiplied, became bilateral, spreading to both her arms and elbows. Pain became very severe after a neck manipulation. A homoeopath rubbed her arms with oils and ice until they were sore. Her initial treatment was six months of unhelpful physiotherapy with ice packs and pain management training.

The rehabilitation doctor diagnosed her pain in terms of 'synovial thickening' and 'tenderness of the left metacarpo-phalangeal joint and epicondylitis of the wrist extensors and fibrositis of the neck, shoulder down the rhomboids'.

The radiologist saw 'oedema of the biceps tendon' on ultrasonography. Another rheumatologist opined that 'the primary condition is osteo-arthritis of the hands afflicting in particular the first carpo-meta-carpo joint as well as the distal terminal interphalangeal joints of the fingers' and deemed it 'consistent with mild RSI'.

An EMG report suggested 'bilateral ulnar nerve lesions at the elbow', a surprising finding in view of her complaint of pain in her thumb (that is, on the wrong side of her hand for it to be attributed to ulnar nerve involvement). Another EMG led to diagnosis of 'findings consistent with right CTS' and, at one stage, she seemed to be convinced of the need for CTR but she did not pursue it.

An unrelated ganglion was noted but she had made no complaint about it.

Neck manipulation had left Mrs Fritz with a new and long-lasting problem: a stiff, sore neck and symptoms which one doctor, later in the proceedings, suggested represented 'cervical neuralgia'. Laser machines were not helpful, nor were wax baths or interferential electrotherapy. Unsuccessful therapies had included acupuncture, naturopathy, sometimes iced and sometimes hot water, rubbing till her arms were sore, neck traction, nonsteroidal anti-inflammatory drugs and pain killers. Cervical spine x-rays demonstrated 'osteoarthritic changes with disc space narrowing at the fifth and sixth and sixth and seventh disc spaces and moderate osteo-arthritis of the first metacarpo-phalangeal joint'. Earlier diagnoses had included tenosynovitis, RSI, fibrositis, epicondylitis, consequence of osteopathic manipulation, bilateral ulnar nerve lesions at the elbow, carpal tunnel syndrome, osteoarthritis of metacarpo-phalangeal joint, ganglion and brachial neuralgia.

Mrs Fritz had returned to work when she still had two toddlers at home. Over the next 18 months she claimed time off work with RSI several times until, she said, she was sacked. She had told various people, including the company doctor, that she was not yet ready to go back to work on account of symptoms.

Mrs Fritz moved into the house that she and her husband had been engaged in building while she was becoming symptomatic and the move upset her baby-sitting arrangements with her mother. Then she had her third child. She continued to litigate and continued to report symptoms to medical examiners, arguing that 'I have a permanent injury and I will be unable to do physical work again and, secondly, I'm not educated to do anything else' and 'if it hadn't happened, I'd still be working, of course'. The claimant took the position that her condition could not be caused by anything other than work. I called this nothing/pure hysteria, but a review of her various actions suggests more consciously motivated action.

CASE NUMBER 26

Mrs Green, a 27-year-old assistant manager in a computer company, had been absent from work only for a matter of days or weeks and had already returned.

When she developed pain in both hands she saw a doctor who interpreted her chubby hands as 'swollen' as she had gained a great deal of weight. She took a week off. Voltarin, an anti-inflammatory drug, was said to be helpful for a while and she only took it occasionally. Then she had massage and muscular therapy and hydrotherapy from an alternative healing centre. Her doctors had given her laser therapy, which was ineffective.

A major assignment for her tertiary course was due at the time and this kept her very busy. Mrs Green complained that, as well as working full-time, she had to work on Saturdays and Sundays for no extra pay. She was told that she had RSI at work but it did not affect her at home, typing her assignments. Situational tension myalgia was an acceptable diagnosis and she was very happy to take advice to listen to the signals of her body and to go back to work.

CASE NUMBER 28

Mrs Harapoulos, a 28-year-old Islander who worked as a cleaner, had been absent from work for 18 months and had not returned. 'My hand was very painful,' she said, indicating her left shoulder, 'fingers all numb and I kept dropping things.' After she left work, her symptoms became bilateral, involving her right arm and hand, her left shoulder, her right leg and inside of her foot. She attributed them to her cleaning duties.

An early but unsuccessful CTR on the left side was followed by unspecified pills. Following an X-ray for her shoulder, she reported that her doctor said, 'You will be like that all the time'. Mrs Harapoulos felt that ultrasound, which is a diagnostic procedure, helped her shoulder, in which she had a painful arc. She had nearly got an ulcer from tablets, which were almost certainly non-steroidal anti-inflammatory drugs.

Her marriage had failed after two years. She had only a temporary visa when she married. Mrs Harapoulos had first become ill with abdominal pain, which was investigated, then with the undiagnosable arm pains and depression. When I saw her, she was in the process of a divorce, living in a boarding house, while her former husband was borrowing money to get their house finished and ready to sell as everything she had earned was invested in it. This was functional disorder, somatization of distress and depression.

CASE NUMBER 51

Mrs Jones, a 35-year-old process worker in a tile factory, had been absent from work for 24 months and had not yet returned. Her arm symptoms came on at work as if they were a continuation of normal occupational fatigue. Physiotherapy was unsuccessful, as were ultrasound, pills, rest, time off work, a splint that she liked, non-steroidal anti-inflammatory drugs, the application of ice and, at other times, the application of heat. She was to be assessed for rehabilitation. She believed that she had RSI, a ganglion, the vague consequences of a fall, CTS, shoulder problem, peri-arthritis.

Retrenchments were imminent in her workplace. Mrs Jones went off with RSI and continued to receive income in the form of workers' compensation long after everyone else had been laid off. After she had gone off work she had become totally incapacitated and unable to cope at home, where she had previously been house-proud. She attracted a diagnosis of major depression, with functional disorder. Mrs Jones had not been so depressed when she went off work. She had no workplace to which to return.

CASE NUMBER 54

Ms King, a 36-year-old VDU operator, had been absent from work for 36 months and had not returned. She was put off work for three days when a pain in the wrist came on during a period of overtime. The pain progressed all of a sudden to the shoulder, around the neck, down both arms and across the chest.

Her family doctor was aware of the emotional origins of her complaints so Ms King changed to another. This doctor referred her to a specialist, who advised her that she would have to give up VDU work. Neck traction was started but that was described as 'hopeless' and she reported that 'everything that they have done has made me worse'. Ms King had not used her left arm at all at work and had been away from work for a long time when splints were prescribed for each arm. She was also prescribed antidepressants, but in sub-therapeutic doses as this treatment was fashionable for pain and promoted by pharmaceutical companies. She thought that she had RSI attributed to keyboard work, or a neck problem.

Ms King was an unlucky woman who had a difficult life. A hysterectomy when she was 29 had left her childless. She divorced, then won the lottery but subsequently lost all the money. She was embroiled in a family feud. Her sister dealt punitively with her attempt to reconcile with her brother. Ms King had started to misuse alcohol and had made two suicide attempts. Her GP had sent her for treatment but she phoned to say that her solicitor was unhappy about her seeing me and she cancelled further appointments. The precipitating stress had been the breakdown of a significant relationship. This was somatized depression, functional disorder.

CASE NUMBER 56

Mrs Loucas, a 37-year-old clerk, had been absent from work for 11 months and had not returned. She was typing one day and her left arm just started hurting. She thought that she had a viral illness with aches and pains, so she attended her doctor. He told her that it was due to computers. Her history was given in a melodramatic way and it left me with the impression that she was not familiar with her own symptoms but very familiar with the literature on RSI. She reported thus:

> Oh God, I would dearly love to work. I am sick and tired of staying home, but I get a sore arm. I try not to use it. I would dearly love to work but I am trying not to use my arm. It feels weak and I'm relying on my right arm and, you know. I'm using the right arm too often. As I said before, is it called RSI? Repetitive? What did they call it? Oh God, can't even think of its name, it's some strain. They said it could only be because of using the computer. You know it's frightened me. I wish I could do work, [sigh] I feel like I'm restricted.

Mrs Loucas gave this account in terms of what the doctor had said. 'The GP said I needed physio.' The physiotherapist gave ultrasound, which 'helped a little bit', and hot packs, which 'really helped'. Splinting her hand with a scarf also 'really helped'. Pills were prescribed but were unhelpful. She told me that a specialist had said that it was all due to computers and that her symptoms were consistent with this kind of injury. One doctor suggested 'cervical spondylosis, at C5/6 and 6/7'. I thought she was acting out the role of a victim and this was consistent with her histrionic traits.

CASE NUMBER 68

Mrs Murphy, a 41-year-old typist, had been absent from work for nine months and had not returned.

'When my doctor told me that I had RSI, I was devastated,' she told me, 'I had thought that my neck and back ache were caused by a virus.' Her symptoms got worse immediately after the diagnosis was made: the next day she had pains from the wrists up and the day after that she could not do input work on the computer.

An occupational therapist told her that the she had needed a foot rest, rest and physiotherapy. Mrs Murphy had electrical (perhaps conductivity) tests. Her neck was manipulated, splints were suggested for her wrists. Non-steroidal anti-inflammatory drugs and other medications were ineffective. Multiple sites of origin were suggested and multiple therapeutic interventions were offered but declined. Neck traction was tried without success. She was re-educated in how she might reduce how fast she worked and advised to go back on restricted duties.

During her marriage, Mrs Murphy had hardly worked at all and she had no economic motivation to work. Her husband was already retired. She had been offered part-time work by a relative and then she became outraged because he wanted her to work full time. She bad-mouthed her employer. I later learnt, from an unexpected source, of her husband's concurrent litigation for his occupational problems and the many problems within the family. This was one of the three cases where no stressor was identified at interview. Mrs Murphy seemed to be acting with the collusion of her doctor and she knew enough not to tell me everything.

CASE NUMBER 71

Mrs Nolan, a 41-year-old clerk, had been absent from work for 11 months and had already returned. No stressors were identified.

A lump in her upper arm was identified in the course of a consultation for contraceptive advice. She had an underlying shoulder problem that might have developed in the course of her work, which required her to reach behind her. The doctor had been injecting steroids into her shoulder. A muscle swelling, said to have been 'the size of an egg', had developed near the insertion of the deltoid muscle and the lump under her armpit was thought to be an abscess.

Mrs Nolan had a traumatic disease, a shoulder problem with an infection apparently caused by the injection into it. She would have continued to work with her sore shoulder problem but had to take time off, on compensation, as a result of the treatment.

CASE NUMBER 72

Mrs Origan, a 41-year-old machinist, had been absent from work for over five years and had not returned. Pain started in her right hand, then in her left hand, her arm and her shoulder. She blamed her machine.

Full investigation revealed anaemia of gynaecological origin. She reported her doctor as saying, 'You will never work again'. Mrs Origan was given a collar, an orthopaedic pillow and sent for physiotherapy. She was given a Cybex test, said to identify motivation and she sabotaged it, faking weakness. Each fortnight, she attended a workers' health clinic, where a doctor told her that he found virtually all of her muscles to be tender and diagnosed overuse syndrome, RSI and inflammation. She was prescribed a left Futuro splint and told to apply ice. The doctor told her that a return to work would cause an exacerbation of her condition.

Another doctor wrote that she had soft tissue damage to the scapular area and her deltoid. Another saw 'disc narrowing at fifth to sixth level and a slight kyphosis'. She developed epigastric pain from non-steroidal anti-inflammatory drugs and aspirin. She was also using benzodiazepines.

Before she reported arm and shoulder symptoms, Mrs Origan had been sick for four years with some other problems. At the height of the epidemic, there were about 50 other cases at her workplace. She tried to tell me that she had never heard of RSI, but when that was questioned she confessed that she knew 'just one girl'. She had iron deficiency anaemia and the doctor sent her to a gynaecologist for a hysterectomy. This was undertaken while she was on compensation for RSI and tenosynovitis.

Her presentation was well rehearsed. When Mrs Origan reported her initial symptoms, four years before this consultation, she was still grieving the death of her father. When she went off work she was either still pregnant or had just miscarried. Mrs Origan was very suspicious of me at interview. This seemed to be functional disorder, secondary to general health impairment. The moral aspect of this case was that it provided grounds for exemption from work and four years on compensation.

CASE NUMBER 81

Mrs Peters, a 43-year-old home-care aide, had been absent from work for 42 months and had not returned.

She woke up one night with her whole right hand feeling big, heavy and numb. She thought she had been lying on her arm. She went to an emergency department in the morning. Tenosynovitis was diagnosed and a certificate was provided. Symptoms spread involving her whole hand to the top of her wrist, extending up her forearm into the elbow and ultimately involving her neck. Mrs Peters developed weakness, paresis, inability to pick up a plate, shooting pains and inco-ordination.

A splint was prescribed to use only at night, as well as rest in conjunction with time off on compensation. Non-steroidal anti-inflammatory drugs were unsuccessful, as were physiotherapy, nerve stimulation, ultrasound, heat and ice treatments. Pain recurred if she tried to do anything. An arthroscopic examination of her wrist was reported as having shown inflammation. An RSI clinic provided rehabilitation, which consisted, in part, of doing crafts with a group of women similarly affected.

Her two daughters had completed university and school just as she went off work on compensation. Mrs Peters was disingenuous when she told me she had never heard of RSI or teno, as her presentation made it obvious that she was very familiar with the literature of preventing RSI or, perhaps, had been educated in the jargon by a friend or a clinician using a checklist. No precipitating stress was identified, but depression seemed to predate the onset of physical symptoms and remained an ongoing problem. This was coded functional disorder, because she was clinically depressed.

CASE NUMBER 82

Mrs Quinn, a 44-year-old secretary, had been absent from work for ten months and had not returned.

'I just mentioned in passing that my wrists were paining,' she told me, 'so he put me off.' She attributed the symptoms to her visual display screen being of the wrong height for her, so she had to put it up on a telephone book. As further proof of her entitlement to this claim, she cited a manufacturer of ergonomic furniture who had been called in to solve the RSI problem in her office. He told me, 'It's the way the keyboard is made. It's not horizontal. It's higher at the back and lower at the front. This gives you RSI.'

On doctor's instructions, she had tried swimming but, on the third day, she couldn't move her arms. Mrs Quinn had suffered from excessive fatigue for several years and had identified with having chronic fatigue syndrome.

It was apparent from her presentation that she believed her employer would have a strong case to answer because the furniture salesman equated bad furniture with cause and this legitimated her continuing problem.

Mrs Quinn failed to reveal to me or to anyone else that she had arranged to adopt a five-year-old girl. She took a certificate for compensation and immediately went overseas to pick up the child while receiving payments. She withheld information about this child for the greater part of the second interview, until I asked her who was the small child who had been with her in the waiting room of another doctor. That doctor had noted that a child accompanied Mrs Quinn and she had to tell me after that. This information would never have reached me otherwise. The insurer did not know about her adoption of the child.

Mrs Quinn claimed to like her boss, but she repeated a number of malicious things that other girls had told her of him. She scored over 61 on the Zung Depression Scale, on which a score of 56 would suggest severe depression. She didn't look at all depressed. I could not classify this material, as her presentation included many malingering indicators.

CASE NUMBER 83

Ms Robinson, a 44-year-old trade skill teacher and a supervisor, had been absent from work for nine months and had not returned.

Ms Robinson came back from her holidays and presented her paralysed arm. Overuse was diagnosed to account for the monoplegia. Her work included snipping off loose threads with special scissors. She volunteered:

I didn't think there was anything seriously wrong with my arm, but the doctor says I need treatment and he read me some case histories reporting what happened where people have been overused. I believe that. I have no reason to believe anything else.

Unsuccessful therapies included rest, time off activity, acupuncture, splinting, machines at the physiotherapist's and cortisone injections, non-steroidal anti-inflammatory drugs, laser therapy TENS machine and a heavy brace for her elbow. She believed that she was suffering from Stage III RSI and overuse causing inflammation, but why an overuse syndrome might have affected her after her vacation remained unanswered.

Her mother, who lived nearby, had become increasingly sick with heart disease and Ms Robinson either wanted to or was obliged spend more time with her. She argued strenuously against the proposition that she should delegate the chore of snipping off loose threads and get on with teaching and supervising. This seemed to be a conflict neurosis, generated by Ms Robinson's conflict between working and attending her sick mother's needs, but there were malingering indicators as well.

CASE NUMBER 98

Mrs Stevens, a 55-year-old process worker involved in the manufacture of switchboards, had been absent from work for 42 months and had not returned.

Her symptoms started with non-recovering tiredness, a sore neck and soreness in the arms below the elbow. All this gradually progressed to her shoulders and she presented with the loss of sensibility to pinprick in her face as well as her arms.

'If it persists,' her doctor told her, 'you will have it for the rest of your life.' Her specialist diagnosed flexor tenosynovitis and found evidence of carpal tunnel syndrome together with 'chronic overuse regional neck arm pain' and, later, 'chronic pain triggered by tissue damage', which her doctor reported on, saying that this 'can represent a "neuro-psychological" event in the same category as anxiety and depression, with each emotional state having neuro-chemical correlates that are being increasingly defined'.

The thermography centre reported that re-warming of her right palm after having put it in cold water was abnormal.

Mrs Stevens' symptoms were bilateral and involved her entire arms, neck and shoulders, not only the territory of the median nerve. A carpal tunnel release on one wrist was unsuccessful, her symptoms returned and she did not ever go back to work. The doctor who had recommended CTR later noted that Mrs Stevens had hypaesthesia (lack of feeling) to pinprick in both hands in a glove distribution, some dullness to pinprick of her face and general weakness of her grip.

She eventually settled for regular appointments with a known RSI sympathiser who perceived her problems in terms of overuse and sympathetic nervous system problems. According to another surgeon, she had chronic tenosynovitis affecting both arms and a 20 and 25 per cent impairment, or loss of use. He also added 'mild cervical spondylitis' and then 'gross functional overlay' to his description. (Impairment translates into money in common law claims.)

Mrs Stevens thought what was wrong with her was 'my muscles', that the doctors had said 'muscles or, of course, teno'. Mrs Stevens brought in an array of unused and old bottles of pills and potions, non-steroidal anti-inflammatory drugs, codeine phosphate and a bottle of Indospray two years old.

A claim for work disability had been lodged just after she had paid the final mortgage payment on her house. Her husband was simultaneously granted the invalid pension. If she had continued to work, his pension would have been reduced at a dollar-for-dollar rate above a certain very low threshold.

It would have been senseless for her to continue to work as her income would have been reduced effectively by half. She had also lodged a claim at common law.

CASE NUMBER 99

Ms Thompson, a 57-year-old process worker involved in the pharmaceutical industry, had been absent from work for 26 months and had not returned

A year before she went off work she had some symptoms. One day she was having trouble keeping up with her machine, and her supervisor, on learning that she was having trouble with her hands, told her to see a doctor. Ms Thompson attended a designated workers' clinic at a teaching hospital, where she was put off work. Her extensive education about RSI was evidenced by her recitation of RSI theory during her consultation.

Pain eventually settled in the thumb, which the doctor injected. At one stage, her complaint was that when she carried her shopping in her right hand she got numbness in the index, middle and ring fingers, going up her arm and crossing to the right side of the base of her skull. She also got these symptoms when carrying a single loaf of bread. Symptoms in a glove distribution of numbness and insensitivity to pinprick involved the base of her thumb and later spread to the centre of her palm. CTR was suggested.

Non-steroidal anti-inflammatory medication was ineffective but she liked a popular over-the-counter analgesic at night.

While receiving compensation, Ms Thompson was occupied as a baby sitter for her grandchild. This freed the child's mother, with whom she was living, to work. She was hoping for reconciliation with her long-estranged husband. Ms Thompson had come back to work late in life and she had been indoctrinated into a strong belief in the dangers of repetitive work. She volunteered that she had been injured, first, by the movement that she performed and, second, by staying in the same position for too long. This seemed to be pure hysteria/nothing at all as she resolved a family problem by entering the compensable sick role.

GLOSSARY

ablate a medical euphemism for destroy.

aetiology medical causation, which is seen as multi-factorial.

algodynia (allodynia) an unusual word for pain seen in Australian medical reports concerning RSI.

algodystrophy (allodynia) unusual words for painful wasting.

arthritis inflammation of a joint.

asymptomatic neither displaying nor causing symptoms.

ataxia lack of co-ordination, inco-ordination.

brachial plexus a network of interlacing nerves composed of the lower four cervical and the first thoracic, located in the neck and armpit and emerging as the nerves that supply the arm.

butazolidine an old-fashioned, but effective, anti-inflammatory medicine.

carpal tunnel release surgery to decompress the medial nerve in the carpal tunnel.

carpal tunnel syndrome symptoms in the territory of the median nerve consequent on compromise of the median nerve in the carpal tunnel. See compression neuropathy.

causalgia a burning pain sometimes caused by injuries to nerves with changes to be seen in the affected parts.

compression neuropathy the peripheral symptoms attributable to a compression of a nerve anywhere along its path.

conversion (conversion hysteria) refers to changing of emotions into symptoms in the body. See hysteria.

cultural iatrogenesis iatrogenesis induced by cultural beliefs.

cumulative trauma disorders the American name for repetitive strain injuries, referring to any number of conditions presumptively caused by trauma.

de Quervain's disease tenosynovitis of the extensor brevis and abductor longus tendons of the thumb.

disc lesion problem with a prolapsed or decayed inter-vertebral disc.

disease untoward changes in the body, the sum total of one or more pathological processes.

dys- (prefix) bad, hard or difficult.

dystonia abnormal tone in muscles. It can be spastic, meaning tight, or flaccid, meaning limp.

endemic present in the community at all times but occurring only in small numbers.

epicondylitis inflammation at the epicondyle, thought to occur at the junction of the tendons and bone so it can be at the inside or the outside of the elbow.

epidemic occurring in great numbers.

epistemology the study of the theory of knowledge, or the origins of an idea.

ergonomics the study of work.

extensor tenosynovitis inflammation of the sheaths of the tendons that straighten the fingers.

flexor tenosynovitis inflammation of the sheaths of the tendons that bend the fingers and wrist.

frozen shoulder a general term referring to limitation of movement of a shoulder. It can have a number of causes and pathologies.

functional overlay the presence of symptoms over and above those caused by the lesion or disease and presumed to have emotional causes.

functional the most common medical use implies the absence of an organic base for a disorder of function. When a physician says that someone has a 'functional disorder' it implies the absence of pathology. 'Functional' sometimes implies psychogenesis, possibly a neurosis, or a somatization symptom. In sociology and psychology, 'functional' implies lack of disadvantage. The many people with 'functional disorder' in this epidemic were having, sociologically speaking, 'functional' reactions.

furphy a rumour, term derived from a mobile water tank made by the Furphy family of Shepparton, Victoria.

hysterical personality see histrionic personality disorder.

histrionic personality disorder a personality type characterised by attention-grabbing, dramatic shallow emotions that can change rapidly. A histrionic presentation is broad-brushed and devoid of detail.

iatrogenesis the unintentional causing of a disease or symptoms through a physician's actions or words. It is clinical when pain, sickness or death result from the provision of medical care; it is social when health policies reinforce or generate dependency and ill health; and it is structural when medically sponsored behaviour and delusions restrict the vital autonomy of people by undermining their confidence in growing up, caring for each other and aging.

idiopathic referring to a pathology or cause that is not known.

illness a state or status accorded to a person who feels unwell.

Index Medicus an annual summary of the published medical literature. There is a five-yearly cumulative index of publications and a citation index, which records how frequently others have referenced an item.

intersection syndrome a name given to a set of continuing symptoms where release of presumed de Quervain's syndrome has failed to relieve them.

kyphosis curvature of the spine going forward.

medicalisation the process of deeming a behaviour or subject to be within the clinical jurisdiction of the medical profession.

morbus an obsolete term for disease.

necrosis the pathological death of a group of cells or tissue.

neuropathy a pathology of nerves, for example, peripheral, toxic, compression or entrapment neuropathy.

neurosis originally, a set of symptoms for which no physical cause can be found, that is, hysteria. At the turn of the twentieth century, as the mental causes became evident, the term evolved to psychoneurosis, then neurosis, which in turn became more specific as its form and contexts were tagged on, as in anxiety, conflict, combat, compensation, occupational, traumatic or war neurosis. The term is currently out of fashion.

nocebo an anti-placebo, a communication or remedy that has the effect of making a patient sicker.

occupational cramp another name for occupational neurosis. Other synonyms are anapeiratic paralysis, Beschäftigungneurosen, copodyscinesia (from the Greek words for weariness, difficult motion) craft palsy, cheirospasmus, chorea scriptorum, craft neurosis, crampe des écrivains, crampe télégraphique, fatigue disease, Fingerkrampf, functional spasm, graphospasmus, Kavierkrampf, loss of grip, professional dyscinesiae, paralysis notorarium, le mal télégraphique, mogigraphia, nervose co-ordinatrice des professions, professional impotence, professional hyperkinesis, Schreibekrampf, scrivener's palsy, steel pen palsy and literally hundreds of both specific and archaic occupational cramps and palsies.

occupational neurosis a set of functional symptoms, which occur in a limb or body part used in an occupational task. Occupational neuroses affect the eyes, tongue and legs, as well as arms.

overuse a term never defined but presumed to be the cause of RSI, a synonym for RSI.

palsy paralysis. This word is not generally used for paralysis of organic origin, but tends to refer more to weakness.

paraesthesia a unnatural sensation such as tingling, pins and needles, ants crawling (formication), or of being swollen or burning.

pathology the study of disease at a macroscopic, microscopic or biological level.

pathophysiology abnormal physiology.

pisiform a small bone in the wrist.

placebo an inactive remedy prescribed for any number of reasons, usually for the purpose of humouring the patient.

psychogenesis the causation of symptoms by events in the mind, beliefs, needs, desires and emotions.

psychogenic originating in the mind, hence out of beliefs, emotions and desires.

psychotherapy treatment by the mind, designed to change mental content, which is problematic in causing dysfunction.

psychotropic exerting an effect on the mind.

radial nerve a nerve supplying the hand and arm on the side of the thumb.

rational choice theory a social theory that purports to explain actions by reference to opportunities, beliefs and desires of individuals.

Raynaud's disease intermittent vascular spasm in digital arteries.

reflex sympathetic dystrophy a rare response to injury of nerves of obscure origin, thought to be mediated by the sympathetic nervous system.

repetitive strain injury (RSI) Australian interpretation of epidemic occupational neurosis imputing a hypothetical 'injury' and a presumed cause, 'repetitive strain'.

Scheuermann's osteochondritis a pathology of the vertebral epiphyses of children.

scoliosis curvature of the spine going sideways.

shoulder–hand syndrome disorder of arm characterised by pain and stiffness in the shoulder and a sore hand on the same side, sometimes occurring after myocardial infarction, but having some other causes.

sick role a term from the work of sociologist Talcott Parsons (1951), who described in an idealised way how sick people behaved in the middle of the twentieth century.

somatization the process of experiencing emotions such as distress, anxiety and depression as symptoms in the body, the soma.

somatize o experience stress or anxiety as a feeling in the body, a physical symptom.

stenosis narrowing or contraction of a body, passage or opening.

stereotactic surgery surgery performed with instruments guided in two or three dimensions by a stereoscope. Thalotomy and prefrontal topectomy are procedures that involve cutting or destroying brain tissue.

synovial fluid the fluid produced by the synovium, the lining of a joint or tendon, resulting in a swelling that fluctuates.

tenosynovitis inflammation of the synovial sheath that surrounds a tendon.

tenotomy cutting tendons.

thoracic outlet syndrome a condition caused by pressure on the brachial plexus.

type I error a mistake of failing to diagnose a disease or condition that is present in the patient

type II error a mistaken diagnosis of a condition that is not present in the patient.

ulnar nerve the nerve that supplies the inner side of the arm and the little finger and part of the next.

BIBLIOGRAPHY

Abell P (1996) Sociological theory and rational choice theory. In Bryan Turner (ed.) *The Blackwell Companion to Social Theory*. Blackwell Publishers Ltd, pp. 252–77.

Althaus J (1870) *On scrivener's palsy and its treatment by galvanisation of the cervical sympathetic nerve*. Wertheimer, London.

American Psychiatric Association (1980) *Diagnostic and Statistical Manual of Mental Disorders*. (3rd edn.) American Psychiatric Association, Washington DC.

—— (1987) *Diagnostic and Statistical Manual of Mental Disorders*. (3rd rev. edn.) American Psychiatric Association, Washington DC.

—— (1994) *Diagnostic and Statistical Manual of Mental Disorders*. (4th edn.) American Psychiatric Association, Washington DC.

Anonymous (1972) Writers' cramp [editorial]. *British Medical Journal* 1: 67–68.

Anonymous (1982) *Tenosynovitis and Other Occupational Over-Use Injuries*. Workers' Health Centre, Sydney.

Anonymous. (1982) Writers' cramp [editorial]. *Lancet* 2(8305): 969.

Anonymous (1985) RSI, or "kangaroo paw" [letter]. *Medical Journal of Australia* 142: 423–24.

Appignanesi L, Forrester J (1992) *Freud's Women*. Weidenfeld and Nicholson, London.

Arksey H (1994) Expert and lay participation in the construction of medical knowledge. *Sociology of Health and Illness* 16: 448–68.

Armstrong T, Chaffin D (1979) Carpal tunnel syndrome and selected personal attributes. *Journal of Occupational Medicine* 21: 481–86.

Arndt B (1986) *RSI Explained*. Globe Press, Melbourne.

Asher R (1951) Munchausen's syndrome. *Lancet* 1: 339–41.

Australian Council of Trade Unions (1986) *RSI/Overuse Injuries: Psychiatrists delusions*. (Pamphlet) ACTU, Sydney.

Australian Public Service Association (1984) Australian Public Service Association repetition strain injury campaign: Submission to government. (Text of submission dated 25 September 1984.) *APSA Review* 1(Oct): 47, 49, 51, 53, 237–38.

Awerbuch M (1987a) Repetition strain injuries [letter]. *Medical Journal of Australia* 147: 627–28.

—— (1987b) *RSI: A model of sensory dysfunction: Management of the compensable patient.* Unpublished. 12 August 1987.

—— (1984) Repetition strain injuries. *Medical Journal of Australia* 9: 740–41.

—— (1991) Thermography — its current status in musculoskeletal medicine. *Medical Journal of Australia* 154: 441–44.

Balint M (1957) *Doctor, Patient and Illness.* International Universities Press, New York.

Barondess JA (1979) Disease and illness — a crucial distinction. *American Journal of Medicine* 66: 375–76.

Bawkin H (1945) Pseudodoxia paediatrica. *New England Journal of Medicine* 232: 691–97.

Beard GM (1879) Conclusions from the study of 125 cases of writer's cramp and allied affections. *The Medical Record: The Official Journal of the Association of Medical Record Officers* 224–47.

—— (1880) *A Practical Treatise on Nervous Exhaustion (Neuraesthenia): Its Symptoms, Nature, Sequences, Treatment.* (2nd rev. edn). William Wood, New York.

—— (1881) *American Nervousness: Its Causes and Consequences.* GP Putman, New York.

Becker HS (1963) *Outsiders.* Free Press of Glencoe, New York.

Beech HR (1960) The symptomatic treatment of writer's cramp. In HJ Eysenck (ed.) *Behaviour Therapy and the Neuroses.* Pergamon Press, Oxford, pp. 334–48.

Bell C (1830) *The nervous system of the human body; paper given in 1830.* Washington, 221.

—— (1854) Affection of the voluntary nerves. In *The Nervous System of the Human Body.* Henry Renshaw, London, pp. 436–37.

Bell DS (1989) "Repetition strain injury": an iatrogenic epidemic of simulated injury. *Medical Journal of Australia* 151: 280–84.

Besson JA, Walker LG (1983) Hypnotherapy for writers' cramp [letter]. *Lancet* 1(8314–5): 71–72.

Black P (1987) Psychiatric aspects of regional pain syndrome. *Medical Journal of Australia* 147: 257.

Bloch B (1984) Repetition strain injuries. *Medical Journal of Australia* 140: 684–85.

Bok S (1979) *Lying: Moral Choice in Public and Private Life.* Vintage Books, New York.

Brain RW (1933) Occupational neurosis. In RW Brain (ed.) *Diseases of the Nervous System.* (1st edn.) Oxford University Press, Oxford, pp. 803–06.

—— (1962) Occupational neuroses. In RW Brain (ed.) *Diseases of the Nervous System.* (6th edn.) Oxford University Press, London, pp. 852–54.

Brain RW, Wright AD, Wilkinson M (1947) Spontaneous compression of both median nerves in the carpal tunnel. *Lancet* 1: 277–82.

Bremner B (1985) Union attacks 'peculiar' RSI claims. *Sydney Morning Herald* 25 November.

Brennan P (1985) *RSI: An Explorer's Guidebook.* Primavera Press, Sydney.

Breuer J, Freud S (1955) Studies in hysteria [1893]. In *Complete Psychological Works of Sigmund Freud.* 2. Hogarth Press, London.

Briquet P (1859) *Traité clinique er thérapeutique de l'hystérie.* JB Ballière et Fils, Paris.

Brodie BC (1837) *Lectures Illustrative of Certain Nervous Affectations.* Longman & Co, London.

Brooks PM (1986a) Regional pain syndrome — disease of the eighties. *Post-Graduate Bulletin. Community Medicine. University of Sydney.* 42: 55–59.

—— (1986b) Occupational pain syndromes. *Medical Journal of Australia* 144: 170–71.

—— (1988) Overuse syndrome. *Lancet* 1: 1465.

Browne CD, Nolan BM, Faithfull DK (1984) Occupational repetition strain injuries: Guidelines for diagnosis and management. *Medical Journal of Australia* 140: 329–32.

Budd K (1978) Drugs in the treatment of chronic pain. *Anaesthetics* 33: 531–34.

Burnett I (1925) An experimental investigation into repetitive work. In *Industrial Fatigue Research Board Report No. 30*, HMSO, London.

Canguilhem G (1966) *On the Normal and the Pathological. [1947]* (1978 edn.) D. Reidel, Dordrecht, Holland.

Carter RB (1853) *On the Pathology and Treatment of Hysteria.* John Churchill, London.

Carter SL (1997) *Integrity.* HarperCollins, New York.

Cicourel AV (1973) *Cognitive Sociology.* Penguin, Harmondsworth.

Cleland LS (1987) 'RSI': A model of social iatrogenesis. *Medical Journal of Australia* 147: 238–39.

Cohen ML, Arroyo JF, Champion GD, Browne CD (1992) In search of the pathogenesis of refractory cervicobrachial pain syndrome. A deconstruction of the RSI phenomenon. *Medical Journal of Australia* 156: 432–36.

Collier J, Adie W (1922) Occupation neuroses. In FW Price (ed.) *A Textbook of the Practice of Medicine.* (1st edn.) Oxford University Press, London, pp. 1462–66.

—— (1935) Craft palsy. In FW Price (ed.) *A Textbook of the Practice of Medicine.* (3rd edn.) Henry Frowde and Hodder & Stoughton, London, pp. 1426–27.

Collier J, Adie WJ, Walshe FMR (1937) Craft palsy. In FW Price FW (ed.) *A Textbook of the Practice of Medicine.* (5th edn.) Oxford Medical Publications, London, pp. 1694–98.

Comcare, Australia (1995–96) Annual report, 1995–1996. AGPS, Canberra.

Commissioner for Employees' Compensation (1985–86) Annual Report of the Commissioner. In *Office of the Commissioner for Employees' Compensation, 1985–1986.* Canberra.

Cooke J (1992) Cutback on fatal arthritis drugs. *Sydney Morning Herald* 18 November.

Coye MJ, Smith MD, Mazzocchi A (1984) Occupational health and safety: Two steps forward, one step back. In V Sidel, R Sidel (eds.) *Reforming Medicine: Lessons of the Last Quarter Century.* Pantheon Books, New York, 79–106.

Craig TK, Boardman AP, Mills K, Daly-Jones O, Drake H (1993) The South London Somatization Study. I: Longitudinal course and the influence of early life experiences. *British Journal of Psychiatry.* 163: 579–88.

Craig TK, Drake H, Mills K, Boardman AP (1994) The South London Somatization Study. II. Influence of stressful life events and secondary gain. *British Journal of Psychiatry* 165: 248–58.

Creighton WB (1982) Statutory safety representatives and safety committees:

Legal and industrial relations implications. *Journal of Industrial Relations* 24: 337–64.

Creighton WB, Micallef EJ (1983) Occupational Health and Safety as an industrial relations issue: The Rank/General Electric dispute, 1981. *Journal of Industrial Relations* 25: 225–68.

Crisp AH, Moldofsky H (1965) A psychosomatic study of writers' cramp. *British Journal of Psychiatry* 111: 841–58.

—— (1967) Therapy of writer's cramp [review]. *Current Psychiatric Therapies* 7: 69–72.

Crofts N (1986) RSI — how do doctors know? Transcript of program on Occam's Razor. *New Doctor* 40: 12–14.

Cullen W (1769) *Synopsis nosologicae methodicae.* William Creech, Edinburgh.

Culver CM, Gert B (1982) Rationality in medicine. In *Philosophy in Medicine; Conceptual and Ethical Issues in Medicine and Psychiatry.* Oxford University Press, Oxford.

Cumpston A (1981) *Report on Repetition Injury.* Commonwealth Department of Health, Canberra.

Dalton K (1983) *Repetitive Strain Injuries at Work.* Open Channel for the Victorian Trades Hall Council, Melbourne.

dell'Oso AM (1986) Watch out or it will get you. Good Weekend. *Sydney Morning Herald,* 46.

Dennett X, Fry HJ (1988) Overuse syndrome: a muscle biopsy study. *Lancet* 1(8591): 905–08.

Deves L, Spillane R (1989) Occupational health stress and work organization. *International Journal of Health Services* 19: 351–63.

Douglas D (1985) PS union rejects doctor's RSI claims. *The Age* 25 February.

Dressing P (1981) *A Risk Management Approach in Dealing with Repetitive Type Movement Claims.* Melbourne Chamber of Commerce, Melbourne.

Drury B (1985) Psychiatrist's RSI views draw protests. *Financial Review* 20 November.

Duchenne (de Boulogne) (1860) Note sur le spasm functionnel, etc. *Bulletin de Thérapie* 146–50.

Ehrenreich J, Ehrenreich B (1978) Medicine and social control. In J Ehrenreich (ed.) *The Cultural Crisis in Modern Medicine.* Monthly Review Press, New York, pp. 38–79.

Elenor R (1981) *Tenosynovitis and Other Repetition Injuries of the Upper Limb: A report.* NSW Department of Industrial Relations, Central Planning and Research Unit, Sydney.

Elster J (1994) Rational choice theory. In *The Polity Reader in Social Theory.* Polity Press, Cambridge, pp. 121–12:

Elvey RL (1991) The clinical relevance of signs of adverse brachial plexus tension. International Federation of Orthopaedic Manipulative Therapists Congress, 1988:14. Published in *The Neurogenic Hypothesis of RSI and Commentaries.* National Centre for Epidemiology and Population Health Working Paper No. 24. Australian National University, Canberra.

Elvey RL, Quintner JL, Thomas AN (1986) A clinical study of RSI. *Australian Family Physician* 15: 1314–15, 1319, 1322.

Engel GL (1977) The need for a new medical model: a challenge for biomedicine. *Science* 196: 129–36.

Ewan C, Lowy E, Reid J (1991) Falling out of culture: The effects of repetition strain injury on sufferer's roles and identity. *Sociology of Health and Illness* 13: 168–92.

Fabrega H (1990) The concept of somatization as a cultural and historical product of western medicine. *Psychosomatic Medicine* 52: 653–72.

Farrell K (1998) *Post-traumatic Culture: Injury and Interpretation in the Nineties.* The Johns Hopkins University Press, Baltimore.

Federal Occupational Safety and Health Administration (1999) *Draft ergo standards released 1999.* 9(5).

Ferguson DA (1971a) An Australian study of telegraphists' cramp. *British Journal of Industrial Medicine* 28: 280–85.

—— (1971b) Repetition injuries in process operators. *Medical Journal of Australia* 2: 408–12.

—— (1984) The 'new' industrial epidemic [editorial]. *Medical Journal of Australia* 140: 318–19.

—— (1987) "RSI": putting the epidemic to rest [editorial]. *Medical Journal of Australia* 147: 213–14.

Figlio C (1982) How does illness mediate social relations? Workmen's compensation and medico-legal practices, 1890–1940. In P Wright, A Treacher (eds.) *The Problem of Medical Knowledge: Examining the Social Construction of Medicine.* Edinburgh University Press, Edinburgh, pp. 174–224.

Ford CV (1982) *The Somatizing Disorders.* Elsevier Biomedical, New York.

Foster KR, Huber PW (1997) *Judging Science.* The MIT Press, Cambridge MA.

Freidson E (1970) *Profession of Medicine.* University of Chicago Press, Chicago.

Garfinkel H (1956) Conditions for successful degradation ceremonies. *American Journal of Sociology* 61: 420–24.

Gay P (1988) *Freud: A life for our time.* W. W. Norton, New York.

Gehlen F (1977) Towards a revised theory of hysterical contagion. *Journal of Health and Social Behaviour* 18: 27–35.

Gelder M, Gath D, Mayou R (1991) *Oxford Textbook of Psychiatry.* (2nd edn.) Oxford University Press, Oxford.

Gert B. Clouser KD (1986) Rationality in medicine: an explication. *Journal of Medicine & Philosophy* 11: 185–205.

Gittins R (1986) Why NSW can no longer afford the compo lotto. *Sydney Morning Herald* 1 October.

Goldberg D (1992) The management of medical outpatients with non-organic disorders: The reattribution model. In F Creed, R Mayou, A Hopkins (eds.) *Medical Symptoms Not Explained by Organic Disease.* Royal College of Psychiatrists and Royal College of Physicians of London, London.

Goldberg DP, Blackwell B (1970) Psychiatric illness in general practice: A detailed study using a new method of case identification. *British Medical Journal* 1: 439–43.

Goldberg DP, Bridges KW (1985) Somatic presentations of DSM-III psychiatric disorders in primary care. *Journal of Psychosomatic Research* 29: 563–69.

Goldberg DP, Bridges K, Duncan-Jones P, Grayson D (1987) Dimensions of neuroses seen in primary-care settings. *Psychological Medicine* 17: 461–70.

Goldberg DP, Grayson DA, Bridges K, Duncan-Jones P (1987) The relationship between symptoms and diagnosis of minor psychiatric disorder in general practice. *Psychological Medicine* 17: 933–42.

Goode E, Ben-Yahuda N (1994) *Moral Panics.* Blackwell, Oxford.

Gould BN (1956) *Medical Dictionary.* (2nd edn.) McGraw Hill, New York.

Gowers WR (1888) Occupational neuroses. In *A Manual of Diseases of the Nervous System.* Vol. 3. J & A Churchill, London, pp. 656–76.

Great Britain and Ireland Post Office Departmental Committee (1911) *Report on Telegraphists' Cramp.* His Majesty's Stationery Office, London.

Grol R (1981) *To Heal or to Harm: The Prevention of Somatic Fixation in General Practice.* Royal College of General Practitioners, Exeter.

Grundberg AB, Reagan DS (1985) Pathologic anatomy of the forearm: intersection syndrome. *Journal of Hand Surgery — American Volume* 10: 299–302.

Gun RT (1990) The incidence and distribution of RSI in South Australia 1980–81 to 1986–87. *Medical Journal of Australia* 153: 376–80.

Hadler NM (1984) *Medical Management of the Regional Musculoskeletal Diseases.* Grune & Stratton, New York.

—— (1985) The challenge of musculo-skeletal symptoms in the workplace. *Journal of Hand Surgery* 4: 451–56.

—— (1986) Industrial rheumatology: The Australian and New Zealand experiences with arm pain and backache in the workplace. *Medical Journal of Australia* 144: 191–95.

—— (1992) Arm pain in the workplace: A small area analysis. *Journal of Occupational Medicine* 34: 113–19.

—— (1993) *Coping with Arm Pain in the Workplace. Occupational Musculoskeletal Disorders.* Raven Press, New York.

—— (1998) Coping with arm pain in the workplace [review]. *Clinical Orthoptics* (351): 57–62

Hall W, Morrow L (1988) 'Repetition strain injury': An Australian epidemic of upper limb pain. *Social Science and Medicine* 27: 645–49.

Head H (1910) *Albutt and Rolleston's System of Medicine.* (2nd edn.) Macmillan, London.

Henker FO (1984) Psychosomatic illness: Biochemical and physiologic foundations. *Psychosomatics* 25: 19–24.

Hocking B (1987) Epidemiological aspects of "repetition strain injury" in Telecom Australia. *Medical Journal of Australia* 147: 218–22.

—— (1988) Overuse syndrome. *Lancet* 1(8600): 1465.

Hopkins A (1989) The social construction of repetition strain injury. *Australian and New Zealand Journal of Sociology* 25: 239–59.

Howie A, Wyatt A (1985) Profile of an ergonomist. *Journal of Occupational Health and Safety* 1: 154–59.

Hudgson P (1982) Writers' cramp [editorial]. *British Medical Journal* 286: 585–86.

Hunter D (1955) *The Diseases of Occupations.* (1st edn.) English Universities Press, London, pp. 775–81.

—— (1957) *The Diseases of Occupations.* (2nd edn.) The English Universities Press, London, pp. 797–803.

—— (1962) *The Diseases of Occupations.* (3rd edn.) The English Universities Press, London, pp. 850–56.

—— (1969) *The Diseases of Occupations.* (4th edn.) The English Universities Press, London, pp. 880–85.

—— (1971) *The Diseases of Occupations.* (5th edn.) The English Universities Press, London.

—— (1987) *The Diseases of Occupations.* (6th edn.) The English Universities Press, London.

Hunter FJ (1985) Overuse injury (or RSI) — it's been around since Shakespeare's day. *Australian Law News* 20: 28–33.

Huth EJ (1976) Illness. In EJ Cassell (ed.), *The Healer's Art: A new approach to the doctor–patient relationship.* Lippincott, New York, p. 48.

Huxley P, Goldberg D (1975) Social versus clinical prediction in minor psychiatric disorders. *Psychological Medicine* 5: 96–100.

Illich I (1974) Medical nemesis. *Lancet* 1(863): 918–21.

—— (1975) *Limits to Medicine: The expropriation of health.* Penguin Books, London.

Illsley R (1980) *Professional or Public Health? Sociology in Health and Medicine.* The Nuffield Provincial Hospitals Trust, London.

Janet P (1901) *The Mental State of Hystericals: A Study of Mental Stigmata and Mental Accidents.* Putnam, New York.

—— (1925) *Principles of Psychotherapy.* George Allen & Unwin, London.

Jasanoff S (1989) The problem of rationality in American health and safety regulation. In R Smith, B Wynne (eds.) *Expert Evidence.* Routledge, London, pp. 151–83.

Jelliffe SE (1910) *A System of Medicine.* Oxford University Press, London, pp. 786–95.

Joravsky D (1970) *The Lysenko Affair.* Harvard University Press, Cambridge MA.

Kaplan HI, Saddock BJ, Freedman AM (1980) *Comprehensive Textbook of Psychiatry.* Vol. 3. Wilkins and Wilkins, Baltimore.

Katon W, Ries R, Kleinman A (1984) A prospective DSM-III study of consecutive somatization patients. *Comprehensive Psychiatry* 25: 208–15.

Kavanagh J (1984) Keyboard cripples: The avalanche looms. *Business Review Weekly* 13–17 November.

Keikenwan SL (1973) Nihon sangyo-eisei gakkai keikenwan shockogun iinkal hokokusho (Report of the committee on occupational cervicobrachial syndrome of the Japan Association of Industrial Health). *Japanese Journal of Industrial Health* 15: 304–11.

Kendell RE (1975) *The Role of Diagnosis in Psychiatry.* Blackwell Scientific Publications, London.

Kennedy I (1981) *The Unmasking of Medicine.* George Allen & Unwin, London.

—— (1988) *What is a Medical Decision? Treat Me Right: Essays in medical law and ethics.* Clarendon Press, Oxford, pp. 19–21.

Kerckhoff AC, Back KW (1968) *The June Bug: A study in hysterical contagion.* Appleton Century Crofts, New York.

King L (1975) Some basic explanations of disease: An historian's viewpoint. In HT Engelhardt, SF Spicker (eds.) *Evaluation and explanation in the biomedical sciences: Proceedings of the First Trans-disciplinary Symposium on Philosophy and Medicine, held at Galveston, May 9–11, 1974.* Reidel, Dordrecht, pp. 11–27.

Kinnear Wilson S (1941) *Occupation Neuroses. Neurology.* Vol. 11. William Wood, Baltimore.

Kirmayer LJ, Robbins JM (eds.) (1991) *Current Concepts of Somatization: Research and clinical perspectives.* American Psychiatric Association Washington, DC (Spiegel D, ed. *Progress in Psychiatry* Number 31).

Kleinman A (1988) *Rethinking Psychiatry*. The Free Press, New York.

Kleinman A, Kleinman J (1985) Somatization. The interconnections among depressive experiences and the meanings of pain. In A Kleinman, B Good (eds.) *Culture and Depression: Studies in the anthropology and cross-cultural psychiatry of affect and disorder*. University of California Press, Berkeley and Los Angeles.

Kräupl-Taylor F (1976) The medical model of the disease concept. *British Journal of Psychiatry* 128: 588–94.

Kräupl-Taylor F, Scadding J (1980) The concept of disease. *Psychological Medicine* 10: 419–24.

Kuhn TS (1970) *The Structure of Scientific Revolutions*. (2nd edn, enlarged) University of Chicago Press, Chicago.

—— (1974) Second thoughts on paradigms. In F Suppe (ed.) *The Structure of Scientific Theories*. University of Illinois Press, Urbana, 459–82.

Lang A, Sheehy M, Marsden C (1982) Anticholinergics in adult-onset dystonia. *Canadian Journal of Neurological Science* 9: 313–19.

Latour B (1987) Science in Action: How to follow scientists and engineers through society. Open University Press, Milton Keynes.

Lees A, Turjanski N, Rivest J, Whurr R, Lorch M, Brookes G (1992) Treatment of cervical dystonia, hand spasms and laryngeal dystonia with botulinus toxin. *Journal of Neurology (Germany)* 239: 1–4.

Lewis MJ (1886) The neural disorders of writers and artisans. In W Pepper, L Starr (eds.) *A System of Medicine by American Authors*. Sampson Low, Marston, Searle and Rivington, London, pp. 504–43.

Lidcombe Workers' Health Centre (1979) A Critique of Current Legislation and Administration: Submission to the NSW Inquiry into Occupational Health and Safety. Workers' Health Centre, Sydney.

Lipowski ZJ (1968) Review of consultation psychiatry and psychosomatic medicine. III. Theoretical issues. *Psychosomatic Medicine* 30: 395–422.

—— (1986) Somatization, a borderland between medicine and psychiatry. *Canadian Medical Association Journal* 135: 609–14.

—— (1987a) Somatization: Medicine's unsolved problem [editorial]. *Psychosomatics* 28: 294–97.

—— (1987b) Somatization: The experience and communication of psychological distress as somatic symptoms. *Psychotherapy and Psychosomatics* 47: 160–67.

Lishman WA (1980) *Organic Psychiatry: The psychological consequences of cerebral disorder*. Blackwell Scientific Publications, London, pp. 785–89.

Liversedge LA, Sylvester JD (1955) Conditioning techniques in the treatment of writer's cramp. *Lancet* 1: 1147–49.

Lowy AH (1983) Pathogenesis of overuse syndromes affecting the upper limb. *Medical Journal of Australia* 2: 605.

—— (1984) Repetition strain injuries. *Medical Journal of Australia* 1: 605.

Lowy E (1992) *Pilgrimage of Pain* [Doctoral dissertation]. University of New South Wales, Sydney.

Lucire Y (1986) Neurosis in the workplace. *Medical Journal of Australia* 145: 323–27.

—— (1987) Carpal tunnel syndrome [letter]. *Journal of Hand Surgery — American Volume* 12: 483–84.

—— (1988) Social iatrogenesis of the Australian disease 'RSI' [review]. *Community Health Studies* 12: 146–50.

—— (1990) *The Role of the Psychiatric Assessor in Personal Injury Claims*. Presented at RANZCP Forensic Psychiatry Conference, Leura, NSW, November.

—— (1996) *Ideology and Aetiology: RSI: An epidemic of craft palsy*. Doctoral dissertation. University of New South Wales, Sydney.

Mace CJ (1992) Hysterical conversion. I: A history. *British Journal of Psychiatry* 161: 369–77.

—— (1992) Hysterical conversion. II: A critique. *British Journal of Psychiatry* 161: 378–89.

Maeda K (1977) Occupational cervicobrachial disorder and its causative factors. *Journal of Human Ergology* 6: 193–202.

Margolis J (1976) The concept of disease. *Journal of Medicine and Philosophy* 1: 238–55.

Masear VR (1986) Reply to Dr Lucire. *Journal of Hand Surgery* 11: 483–84.

Masear VR, Hayes J, Hyde A (1986) An industrial cause of carpal tunnel syndrome. *Journal of Hand Surgery* 11: 222–27.

Mathews J, Calabrese N (1981) Tenosynovitis and overuse injuries … a plan for action. *Health and Safety Bulletin* 1: 1–37

—— (1982) Guidelines for the prevention of repetitive strain injury (RSI). *Health and Safety Bulletin* 18: 1–33.

—— (1983) ACTU health and safety policy: Prevention of repetitive strain injury. *Health and Safety Bulletin* 29: 1–4.

McEvedy CP, Beard AW (1973) A controlled follow-up of cases involved in an epidemic of 'benign myalgic encephalomyelitis'. *British Journal of Psychiatry* 122: 141–50.

McIntosh P (1986) Grant is a pittance, says volunteer worker. *The Sydney Morning Herald* 8 January.

McPhee B (1980) *Tenosynovitis: The physiotherapist's viewpoint*. Proceedings of the 20th NSW Industrial Safety Convention and Exhibition. Organising Committee, Sydney.

—— (1981) *The Mechanism of Repetition Strains. Seminar on Tenosynovitis*. Manly-Warringah Productivity Group, Sydney.

Meador CK (1965) The art and science of nondisease. *New England Journal of Medicine* 1: 92–95.

Meekosha H (1986) Eggshell personalities strike back — a response to the bosses' doctors on RSI. *Refractory Girl* May: 2–6.

Melzac R, Wall PD (1965) Pain mechanisms, a new theory. *Science* 150: 971–79.

Mempel E, Kucinski L, Witkievicz B. Writers' cramp treated successfully by thalotomy. *Neurol Neurochirug (Poland)* 20: 475–80.

Merskey H (1986) Variable meanings for the definition of disease. *Journal of Medicine and Philosophy* 11: 215–32.

Micale M (1994) On the 'disappearance' of hysteria: A study in the clinical deconstruction of a diagnosis. *Isis* 84: 496–526.

Morris DB (1991) *The Culture of Pain*. University of California Press, Berkeley and Los Angeles.

Morris M, Sharp P (1986) RSI a non diagnosis? Two surgeons tell. *Australian Surgeon* 1: 7–8.

Munro I (1979) *It hurts like hell*. Australian Film and Television School, Sydney.

Murphy M (1989) Somatization: Embodying the problem. *British Medical Journal* 298: 1331–32.

Nathan PA, Meadows KD, Doyle LS (1988) Institution Portland Hand Surgery and Rehabilitation Center, Oregon 97210. Title Occupation as a risk factor for impaired sensory conduction of the median nerve at the carpal tunnel. Comment in: *J Hand Surg [Br]* 1991; 16: 230. *Journal of Hand Surgery — British Volume* 13: 167–70.

National Health & Medical Research Council (1982) *Repetition strain injuries: approved guide to occupational health*. Commonwealth Department of Health, Canberra.

National Occupational Health & Safety Commission (1986) *Repetition Strain Injury (RSI): A report and model code of practice*. AGPS, Canberra.

Navarro V (1976) *The Industrialization of fetishism: A critique of Ivan Illich. Medicine under Capitalism*. Croom Helm, London, pp. 106–18.

Oken D (1961) What to tell cancer patients: A study of medical attitudes. *Journal of the American Medical Association* 75: 1120–28.

Osler W (1892) Professional spasms: Occupation neuroses. In *The Principles and Practice of Medicine*. Young J. Penland, Edinburgh and London, pp. 963–65.

—— (1910) Occupation neuroses. In W Osler, T McCrae (eds.) *Modern Medicine: Theory and practice*. Vol. 7. Lea & Febiger, Philadelphia and New York, pp. 786–95.

Owen RR (1985) Instrumental musicians and RSI. *Journal of Occupational Health and Safety* 1: 135–39.

Paget J (1873) Nervous mimicry of organic disease. *Lancet* 2: 511–13.

Pai MN (1947) The nature and treatment of 'writer's cramp'. *Journal of Mental Science* 93: 68–81.

Parsons T (1951) *The Social System*. Free Press, Glencoe, IL.

Patkin M (1985) Wrist posture and RSI. *Canberra Times* August 7.

Pearce B (ed.) (1982) *Health Hazards of VDTs?* HUSAT, Loughborough.

Perrot JW (1961) Anatomical factors in occupational trauma. *Medical Journal of Australia* 1: 73–75.

Poore GV (1878) An analysis of 75 cases of writer's cramp and impaired writing power. *Transcripts of the Royal Medico-Chirurgical Society* 61: 111–45.

Popper KR (1963) *Conjectures and Refutations: The growth of scientific knowledge*. Routledge & Kegan Paul, London.

Proust M (1921) The Guermantes Way, Vol. 5, Pt 1, Ch 2, In *Remembrance of Things Past*. Translated by R and C Cortie (1988).

Public Service Board (1987) *Census of repetition strain injuries in the Australian Public Service December quarter 1986*. AGPS, Canberra.

—— (1987) *RSI strategies: Report of the group implementing recommendations of the Task Force on Repetition Strain Injuries in the Australian Public Service*. AGPS, Canberra.

Quintner J, Elvey R (1991) *The Neurogenic Hypothesis of RSI and Commentaries*. National Centre for Epidemiology and Population Health Working Paper No. 24. Australian National University, Canberra.

Raffle P, Lee W, McCallum R, Murray R (eds.) (1987) Repeated movements and repeated trauma. In *Hunter's Diseases of Occupations*. (7th edn.) Hodder & Stoughton, London, pp. 620–23.

Ramazzini B (1700; reprinted 1964) *De Morbis Artificum (Diseases of Workers)*. Hafner, New York.

Reid J, Ewan C, Lowy E (1991) Pilgrimage of pain: The illness experiences of women with repetition strain injury and the search for credibility. *Social Science and Medicine* 32: 601–12.

Reynolds JR (1869) Remarks on paralysis and other disorders of motion and sensation dependent on idea. *British Medical Journal* 2: 483–85.

—— (1878) *System of Medicine*. Macmillan, London.

Richmond C (1992) Cases involving 20th-century diseases start landing in British courts [letter]. *Canadian Medical Association Journal* 146: 585–86.

Robens (1970–72) *Report of the Committee on Safety and Health at Work*. HMSO, London.

Robinson M (1986) *The industrial relations of repetition strain injury (RSI)*. BEc thesis. University of Sydney, Sydney.

Rouquier A (1951) Crampe des écrivans parkinsonisme, syndrome anxieuse, Guérison par topectomie préfrontale bilatérale. *Bulletin de la Société médicale Hôpitale de Paris* 67: 65.

Royal Australian College of Physicians (1986) *Fellowship Affairs* July 5.

Russell D (1988) A rejoinder to Dr Lucire. *Community Health Studies* 12: 144–45.

—— (1988) Repetition strain injury and psychiatry. *Community Health Studies* 12: 134–39.

Scheff TJ (1978). Decision rules, types of error and their consequences in medical diagnosis. In D Tuckett, JM Kaufert (eds.) *Basic Readings in Medical Sociology*. Tavistock Publications, London, pp. 245–53.

Schultze A, Jacob H (1988) Catamnesic studies of patients with writers' cramp following inpatient psychotherapy. *Psychiatry, Neurology and Medical Psychology [Leipzig]*.

Seigfreid J, Crowell R, Perret E (1969) The cure of tremulous writers' cramp by stereotactic thalotomy. Case report. *Journal of Neurosurgery* 30: 182–85.

Semple JC, Behan BO, Behan WM (1988) Overuse syndrome. *Lancet* 1(8600): 1464–65.

Sheehy MP, Marsden CD (1982) Writers' cramp — a focal dystonia. *Brain* 105: 461–80.

Shorter E (1992) *From Paralysis to Fatigue: A history of psychosomatic illness in the modern era*. Free Press, New York.

Sicherman B (1977) The uses of a diagnosis: Doctors, patients and neuraesthenia. *Journal of the History of Medicine and Allied Sciences* 32: 33–54.

Sikorski J (1985–86) *The diagnosis and classification of repetitive strain injury*. WorkSafe Australia Grant, 1985/1986 (unpublished).

Smelser NJ (1962) *Theory of Collective Behaviour*. Routledge & Kegan Paul, London.

Smith D (1982) New thoughts on repetition injury. *National Times* 17–23 October.

Smith M, Culpin M, Farmer E (1927) *A Study of Telegraphists' Cramp*. HMSO, London. (Council MR, ed. Industrial Fatigue Research Board; vol. 43).

Solly S (1864) Clinical lectures on scriveners' palsy, or the paralysis of writers. *Lancet* 2: 709–11.

Spillane R, Deves L (1986) RSI: Psychological correlates of RSI reporting. *Journal of Occupational Health and Safety* 4: 21–27.

—— (1987) RSI: Pain, pretence or patienthood. *Journal of Industrial Relations* 29: 41–48.

Stekel W (1943) *The Interpretation of Dreams*. Liveright, New York.

Stevens F, Dawson R (1982) *Damages for the Industrial Injury of Tenosynovitis*. Work Health Co. Pty Ltd, Sydney.

Stevens JC, Sun S, Beard CM, O'Fallon WM, Kurland LT (1988) Carpal tunnel syndrome in Rochester, Minnesota, 1961 to 1980. *Neurology* 38: 134–38.

Stevenson M (1987) Progress in the prevention of repetition strain injuries (RSI). *Journal of Occupational Health and Safety* 3: 265–72.

Stewart D (1990) The changing faces of somatization. *Psychosomatics* 2: 153–58.

Stone WE (1983) Repetitive strain injuries. *Medical Journal of Australia* 2: 616–18.

—— (1984) Occupational repetitive strain injuries. *Australian Family Physician* 13: 681–84.

Storey E (1985) Fluoridation bone and repetitive strain injury. *Medical Journal of Australia* 143: 530.

Strohemeyer (1840) Correspondenzblatt.

Sylvester JD, Liversedge JA (1960) Conditioning and the occupational cramps. In HJ Eysenck (ed.) *Behaviour Therapy and the Neuroses: Readings in modern methods of treatment derived from learning theory.* Pergamon Press, Oxford, pp. 334–48.

Szasz TS (1961) *The Myth of Mental Illness.* Harper-Hoeber, New York.

Task Force (1985) *Repetition strain injury in the Australian Public Service.* AGPS, Canberra.

Taylor DC (1985) The sick child's predicament. *Australian and New Zealand Journal of Psychiatry* 19: 130–37.

Taylor R (1979) *Medicine Out of Control: The anatomy of a malignant technology.* Sun Books, Melbourne.

—— (1981) *Repetition Injury Survey Progress Report.* Australian Public Service Association, Canberra.

Taylor R, Gow C, Corbett S (1982) Repetition injury in process workers. *Community Health Studies* 6: 7–13.

Taylor R, Pitcher M (1984) Medical and ergonomic aspects of a dispute concerning occupation-related conditions in data process operators. *Community Health Studies* 8: 172–80.

Tim R, Massey J (1992) Botulinus toxin therapy for neurologic disorders. *Post Graduate Medicine* 91: 327–32.

Toyonaga K, DeFaria CR (1978) Electromyographic diagnosis of the carpal tunnel syndrome. *Arquivos Neuro-Psiquiatria* 36: 127–34.

Travell JG, Simons DG (1983) *Myofascial Pain and Dysfunction.* Williams & Wilkins, Baltimore.

Turner E (1984) Tenosynovitis is mark of exploitation. *The Age* 20 December.

Union of Concerned Scientists. Junk science, accessed 14 September 2002, <http://www.ucsusa.org/junkscience/whatisjunk.html>.

Verral M (1994) Lack of political will, clinical precision stalls RSI research. *Nature* 371: 8.

Walker J (1979) Tenosynovitis, a crippling new epidemic in industry. *New Doctor* 40: 19–21.

Walshe F (1963) Diseases of the nervous system: Acroparaesthesia and the carpal tunnel syndrome. E. and S. Livingstone, Edinburgh.

Walton J (1977) Occupational neuroses. In J Walton (ed.) *Brain's Diseases of the Nervous System.* (8th edn.) Oxford University Press, London, 1200–02.

—— (1985) Occupational cramps or neuroses. In J Walton (ed.) *Brain's Diseases of the Nervous System.* (9th edn.) Oxford University Press, Oxford, pp. 667–68.

—— (1993) *Brain's Diseases of the Nervous System*. (10th edn) Oxford University Press, Oxford, 408–09.

Waugh A (1986) Kangaroo paw, a wonderful new disease from Australia. *Spectator* 15 November.

Welsh R (1972) The causes of tenosynovitis in industry. *Medical Journal of Australia* 41: 16.

Western Region Centre for Working Women Co-Operative (1983) *They Used to Call It 'Process Workers' Arm': A report on repetition injury amongst women in the manufacturing workforce*. The Co-operative, Melbourne.

Williams TG (1981) *Report of the Commission of Inquiry into Occupational Health and Safety*. The Commission, Sydney.

Willis E (1986) Commentary: RSI as a social process. *Community Health Studies* 10: 210–19.

Windschuttle K (1999) *Foreword to David Stove. Anything Goes*. Macleay, Sydney.

Wolinsky FD (1980) *The Sociology of Health: Principles, professions and issues*. Little, Brown, Boston.

Wootton B, Seal VG, Chambers R (1959) *Social Science and Social Pathology*. George Allen & Unwin, London.

World Health Organization (1992) *International Statistical Classification of Diseases and Related Health Problems*. (10th edn.) World Health Organization, Geneva.

Wright GD (1987) The failure of the 'RSI' concept. *Medical Journal of Australia* 147: 233–36.

Wulff HR (1976) *Rational Diagnosis and Treatment*. Blackwell Scientific, Oxford.

LEGAL CASES

Abalos v Australian Postal Commission (1990) 171 CLR 167 F.C. 90/044.

Bolam v. Friern Hospital Management Committee (1957) 1 WLR 582.

Booth AC. Determination number 327 in the matter of Federated Clerks Union of Australia and the Australian Public Service Association (Fourth Division Officers) and the Treasury and the Public Service Board. Australian Conciliation and Arbitration Commission, 1983.

Commissioner for Government Transport v Adamcik (1961) 106 CLR 292.

Cooper v Commonwealth of Australia. 1987. Supreme Court of Victoria. Unreported.

Daubert v Merrell Dow Pharmaceuticals (92-102), 509 U.S.579 (1993).

Frye v United States 54 App. D.C. 46, 47, 293 F. 1013, 1014 (1923).

Lashford v Plessey, Australia Pty. Ltd. 25 March 1982. Supreme Court of NSW. Roden J. Unreported.

Mughal v Reuters Ltd [1993] IRLR 571.

Susan Maree Cooper and: Commonwealth of Australia No. V88/94 AAT No. 4735 Compensation 9 AAR 542.

Tyrrell v Westpac Banking Corporation District Court Western Australian, 14 December 1992, 2924/1990.

INDEX